HOW TO PREVENT FALLS

Better Balance, Independence and Energy in 6 Simple Steps

By Betty Perkins-Carpenter, Ph.D.
SENIOR FITNESS PRODUCTIONS, INC.
Penfield, New York
www.senior-fitness.com

Published by Senior Fitness Productions, Inc.
1780 Penfield Road
Penfield, New York 14526-2104
www.senior-fitness.com
www.howtopreventfalls.com

Printed in Canada

Fifth Edition

©2006 Betty Perkins-Carpenter, Ph.D.
Second Printing 2011

Library of Congress Catalog Card Number: 89-92153

Editing and Concepts: Wes Fox
Layout and Design: Jeffrey Korn \ Creative
Illustrations: Jim Whiting
Additional illustrations: Dick Roberts

ISBN 0-9621031-6-0

Praise for How To Prevent Falls

"There is no doubt that elderly people can decrease the chance of serious injury and death from falls by taking steps to prevent them. For several years, I have followed a regimen to help prevent falling. Now that I have read Betty Perkins-Carpenter's book, I have also begun the exercises that she describes. I recommend this book to all. It should help significantly in reducing the probability of injury or death from falling."
   – Nobel laureate Dr. Linus Pauling (1901-1994), Linus Pauling Institute of
      Science and Medicine, Palo Alto, CA

"Each morning I stretch in bed and do each exercise 14 times. I find that my equilibrium is so improved, it's remarkable. When I used to get up in the night, I had to touch doors and furniture to be sure I did not fall. After stretching, I'm OK."
   – Betty Davis, former U.S. Army Nurse, WW II

"The book is an informative and immensely practical guide for seniors to achieve better balance through fitness. Realistic goals of exercise are repeatedly stressed throughout the text. There is no claim here of developing senior Olympians, but rather an exercise program designed to avoid falls as well as an emphasis on the strong, positive social consequences of self-confidence induced by balance exercise."
   – William J. Hall, M.D., Director of the Center for Healthy Aging,
      University of Rochester

"I practiced daily relaxing into my chair and bed. One day, I slipped in the shower and landed on the tile floor. I was bruised, but nothing more. I was able to get right up after I fell and go confidently about my day."
   – Charlotte Johnson, student in Betty's exercise class

"I think your book *How To Prevent Falls* is marvelous. I do not think that there is any other book on the market today that even comes close. I am shouting the praise of your book to everyone. The techniques in your book cannot fail but to improve anyone's fitness if given an honest try. I am truly happy I ran across your book. It is a treasure. "
   – Mr. Pat Flowers, volunteer at Detroit, MI senior center

"I have read and practiced Dr. Betty Perkins-Carpenter's *How To Prevent Falls* to prevent catastrophic falls. Her *Stretching In Bed Guide* I have been doing for the past five years, and her book should be a manual for all of us as we walk the tight rope of aging. Let's face it, as we enter the Golden Years, sometimes everything that moves hurts, and what doesn't hurt won't move! Practicing her guidelines lessens our chances of being in the army of over 300,000 who fall to Mother Earth annually."
– Sammy Lee, M.D., Olympic gold medalist, diving (1948 & 1952), Olympic diving coach of Olympic gold medalists, member of the President's Council on Physical Fitness and Sports

"You hold in your hands the culmination of a lifetime's work, study and experience. I have had the privilege to watch the development of the Six-Step Balance System™ over decades, and can enthusiastically endorse its use. The clarity of language, excellent illustrations and design recommend this excellent presentation to both the professional and non-professional reader. Baby boomers take note! Falls and their consequences are a major public health problem. A significant part of the solution lies in these pages!"
– Martin W. Korn, M.D., FAAOS Emeritus

"I really feel secure and my balance has improved so much, I no longer need to use my cane."
– June Curtis, former student of Betty's

"I had a condition that made it difficult for me to lift my arms...and I had difficulty walking because of pain in my back. My doctor and other specialists could not come up with a diagnosis. Fortunately, my sister and brother-in-law came to visit and later sent me a copy of *Stretching In Bed*. The movements seemed easy enough, yet when I wiggled my toes, I felt a sensation in my upper back! I realized that these simple, easy movements were having an effect...I loved that I could do them in bed before trying to get up! The results have been amazing. I'm walking again. I can raise my arms high, and I have muscle strength in my legs and arms that I had lost. So, thank you so much for the work you've done."
– E. Addair, Phoenix, AZ

Dedication

More than 50 years ago, I stepped into a challenging and exciting journey in life. Little did I know at that time that it would evolve into many life-saving episodes among seniors. In recent years, the journey has emerged into the Six-Step Balance System.™

This system literally reflects the significant elements of my entire 50-plus-year career. During this time, many people have touched my life. For this I am grateful. This work is truly the result of the efforts of hundreds of individuals. Grateful acknowledgement and a deep sense of indebtedness are made to them all for recognizing the value of the system. They share knowledge, love, support and compassion for humankind.

To my mentors, my colleagues, my students and especially my daughter, Cheryl Perkins-Orefice, and Mike A. Schum, I dedicate this book.

Notice

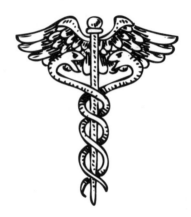

Before you embark on any exercise, activity or program outlined in this book, please be sure to consult your physician. The author and publisher assume no liability in connection with this program.

Contents

WELCOME..1

INTRODUCTION...2

CHAPTER 1
    Stretching in Bed Exercises: Balance System Step 1..................17

CHAPTER 2
    Balance Exercises: Balance System Step 2...................35
        Recommendation #1: Athletic footwear...................44
        Recommendation #2: Constructing a floor balance beam.....61

CHAPTER 3
    Ball Handling Activities: Balance System Step 3.........................79

CHAPTER 4
    Walking while Talking on the Phone: Balance System Step 4.....91
        Recommendation #3: Dressing for comfort..........................97

CHAPTER 5
    The '10 Martini' Slump (The Art of Falling): Balance System
        Step 5...107

CHAPTER 6
    Dancing with a Pillow: Balance System Step 6.........................113

AFTERWORD..120

APPENDIX
    A Contract with Myself..124
    A Checklist for Fall-Proofing Your Home 125
    Important Resources..133

FOOTNOTES...136

ORDER FORM..137

Welcome to How To Prevent Falls

The Six-Step Balance System™

The activities presented in this book are powerful yet simple. The goal of the Six-Step Balance System™ is to help you to prevent falls by practicing and repeating the following exercises on a regular basis. You will strengthen your muscles, increase your confidence and develop an overall sense of well-being.

As you begin using the Six-Step Balance System,™ you will be amazed at the positive results you will soon discover. You will learn how to reduce your fear of falling and, in the event of a fall, learn how to fall more safely. In addition, you will avoid or lessen the chance of serious injury.

Regardless of your physical condition, or how old or young you are, you can achieve maximum benefits by using the Six-Step Balance System.™

The activities
are powerful
yet simple

You'll be
amazed at how
quickly you'll
see results

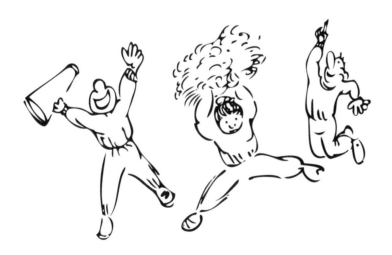

What is the Six-Step Balance System™

The Six-Step Balance System™ is a series of important exercise activities (outlined below) designed to give you the tools to practice fall prevention in the comfort of your own home and at your own pace. Each step of the Balance System™ has its own chapter with easy-to-follow instructions that will carefully guide you step-by-step through each activity. By routinely performing the Six-Step Balance System,™ you will:

- Improve flexibility and mobility by warming your muscles and ligaments while **Stretching in Bed**

- Achieve better posture, increase leg strength, improve confidence and stabilize your entire body through a series of **Balance Activities**

- Discover your body's natural ability to balance, think and move at the same time by performing easy and energizing **Ball Handling Activities**

- Optimize mobility, improve circulation and increase mental alertness by **Walking While Talking on the Phone** (dual tasking)

- Reduce your fear of falling and avoid or limit injury from a fall by practicing the "art of falling" with **The Slump**

- With a soft pillow as a dance partner, learn to move freely, increase energy and improve your balance by **Dancing with a Pillow**

How the Six-Step Balance System™ was created

The Six-Step Balance System™ was developed through many years of research and life-giving experiences. Many talented individuals influenced the overall creation, including physicians, care-providers and seniors themselves. It is also based on my many observations of active young children and athletes who were my students at the Perkins Swim Club (founded in 1964), and my uniquely designed pre-school program for children, ages 2 through 5, where academics were taught through sports and movement, a program known as Fit by Five (founded in 1969).

Developed through many years of research

While serving on the President's Council on Physical Fitness and Sports and as an Olympic diving coach, I recognized the growing need for an effective national fitness program for older adults. As a result, in 1986 I started Senior Fitness to provide guided health and fitness opportunities for seniors. In total, I have worked with older adults in the field of fitness for more than fifty years!

I've worked with seniors for over fifty years

During those years, there were many changes in our society regarding fitness. I learned a great deal about the benefits of good health and why fitness is important. Also, I have witnessed the many problems that can occur with aging. However, it has been my mission to discover fun and effective ways to improve people's lives through innovative fitness activities.

What teaching children about swimming taught me about balance

An important observation that led to the creation of my Six-Step Balance System™ began at my swim club, where we taught children and adults of all ages how to swim and dive.

One of my swimming programs was designed to teach infants how to survive a water accident by rolling over from a face float to a back float in order to breathe. This program was one of the first of its kind in the country, and gained national and international praise when it was made into the best selling video *Born-To-Swim: Together At Home In The Tub*.

It was back in 1964, after studying the video, that I first made the connection between the position of toes and balance. When infants rolled over onto their backs, they were out of balance and their toes were spread wide. When they regained their balance, their toes came back together.

Toes spread wide in order to regain balance

A few years later, the Fit by Five children revealed a similar reaction. When bouncing on a trampoline or walking across a balance beam, some children would lose their balance, and their toes spread wide. When they regained their balance, their toes would return to normal. At that point, I began to understand the relationship between the position of the toes and the ability to balance the body.

During the 1984 Olympic Games in Los Angeles, I studied the toes and balance movements of the Olympic divers. When premier diver Greg Louganis hit his head on the diving board, he had been out of balance and his toes spread.

I was convinced of the connection since I saw it first hand: first in the infant, then in the pre-schooler, and then the skilled Olympic athlete. All had their toes spread while trying to regain their balance, which I later learned was a primitive reflex.

Making this vital connection prompted me to investigate further the physical phenomenon of balance and its role in human fitness activities. Having been an athlete and now, as a fitness instructor, I had a great opportunity to begin to collect and analyze all of the physical data needed to develop and support my new ideas.

I began compiling all the information I had acquired regarding fitness and balance. With this important information, I started using creative body movements and fun activities to teach my students how to regain, improve and maintain their balance.

Making the connection among the infant, adolescent and Olympic athlete

My life's work is translated into the Six-Step Balance System™

Introduction

Fall-related injuries: A growing epidemic

Statistics tell a potentially frightening story

Before we begin the Six-Step Balance System,™ I would like to share some powerful information and statistics concerning falls and related injuries. Truth-of-the-matter is that the act of falling and getting hurt is a major problem for seniors in the United States. The effects are devastating!

The United States Census Bureau predicts that by 2010, the population age 65+ will be 40.2 million. By 2030, that number is expected to reach 71.4 million.[1] A report issued by the U.S. Centers for Disease Control and Prevention states:

- More than one-third of adults ages 65 years and older fall each year.

For those 65+, falls are the leading cause of injury death

- Among people ages 65 years and older, falls are the leading cause of injury deaths and the most common cause of nonfatal injuries and hospital admissions for trauma.

- In 2003, more than 1.8 million seniors were treated in emergency departments for fall-related injuries — more than 421,000 were hospitalized.

- Of all fall-related fractures, hip fractures cause the greatest number of deaths and lead to the most severe health problems and reduced quality of life.

- Only half of older adults who were living independently before their hip fracture were able to live on their own a year later.

- In 2000, direct medical costs totaled *$179 million* for fatal, and *$19 billion* for nonfatal, fall injuries. By 2020, the cost of fall injuries is expected to reach *$43.8 billion.*[2]

Falls are separated into two categories: those caused by environmental factors and those caused by physical factors. The environmental factors, such as poor lighting and slippery floors, etc., are easier to control than physical factors. Physicians at Yale University School of Medicine describe several physical factors that contribute to falling:

- Mental changes (such as cognitive impairment)
- Circulatory, gait or balance problems
- Medication use (particularly sleeping pills)
- Diseases (such as arthritis and osteoporosis)
- Diabetes
- Poor distance vision and muscle weakness[3]

For years, we have felt that falling was part of the aging process. While it is true that aging places some limits on how freely you can move your body, with a little physical fitness you can still increase your chances of moving actively and maintaining good balance.

Falls are separated into two categories

Falling is simply NOT a part of growing older

I have written this book in order to share fun activities for persons of all ages.

I agree with Bob Anderson, a renowned fitness expert, when he says, "All of us have this seemingly miraculous capacity for regaining health, whether it's from something as drastic as surgery, or from poor physical condition caused by lack of activity and bad diet."[4] I know Bob is right. I work with seniors in a variety of settings using the Six-Step Balance System.™ This easy, simple and fun-to-do system really works!

The aging of America brings lots of challenges and opportunities. With people living longer, there will be more and more demands placed on loved ones, Medicare and Medicaid, doctors, insurance companies, hospitals, clinics, nursing homes, churches, community outreach organizations and perhaps other groups whose jobs will be to ensure that lives of seniors are not only extended but are healthy and productive as well.

According to the National Council on Aging, "Every hour one older adult dies from fall-related injuries."[5] To avoid becoming a part of these statistics, I recommend the use of the Six-Step Balance System.™ It is a proven system that could save your life!

How the Six-Step Balance System™ prevents falls

The Six-Step Balance System™ is designed to utilize both a senior's mental and physical condition to help prevent falls. More than being simple "exercises," these brief, targeted activities serve more complex processes that affect the mind and body.

Although the Six-Step Balance System™ is composed of six major steps, the exercises contained in each chapter need not be done in a series or all at once. Nor do they have to be finished completely. The great thing about this system is that it encourages participants to *begin the process* of achieving better balance. Any attempt with any of these exercise activities is a success. The goal is to keep trying different activities as often as you can.

You will train your body to balance safely and move more freely without the fear of falling.

However, we know that accidents can happen no matter how safe we try to make our lives.

By practicing the Six-Step Balance System,™ you will be prepared to fall more safely and gain the confidence to maintain your current lifestyle.

It doesn't matter how much you can do, just start

When a fall is unavoidable, you will be prepared

Introduction

Six-Step Balance System™: Conquer your fear

Fear can affect your quality of life

Internationally known sports psychologist Dr. Alan Goldberg says, "Many people who have fallen or who have seen their friends fall, develop a fear of falling."[6] Once a person becomes afraid of falling, life for that person changes in negative ways, and often causes the person to depend on others to move them from place to place. You have a chance to avoid such conditions by using the Six-Step Balance System.™

During my many years of working with seniors, I've found that their own fears, real or imagined, are the major reasons why they do not exercise and keep moving. Even when it comes to using the Six-Step Balance System,™ some fear they might overdo it, or break something! Many seniors feel that moving an area of the body, which may already be weakened or strained, could make things worse. Some even believe that it would be better not to move the weakened or strained body part than to move it and cause more problems.

Fear can be a BIG BULLY!

There is no question about it, fear can be a big bully, especially after a fall! The result of falling is pain. It's no wonder that after a fall, fear makes many seniors feel like they can never move safely again. At that point, even thinking about falling is scary. Also, as people grow older, they tend to walk very slowly and hold their bodies very rigidly. Remember, a stiff body breaks, a limp body bends.

Dr. Goldberg goes on to say, "Fear may be caused by not knowing what your body is doing in space." The Six-Step Balance System™ will enhance your spacial awareness and will also improve eye, hand and foot coordination and gross motor skills.

In fact, the time it takes to react to things and situations around you will also improve! With the right amount of determination and practice, you can meet your fears head-on and overcome them! What you once thought was impossible to do, will become easy and FUN!

You will enjoy the freedom of moving both indoors and outdoors. In fact, the more time you put into the physical activities that scare you, the less scary they become. You will quickly realize that you have conquered your fears!

As a final word for this section of the book, we must all remember that we cannot guarantee that we will never have an accident or prevent every fall. However, by using the Six-Step Balance System,™ we can be physically and mentally prepared for falling more safely.

Remember, safe adults are no accident!

Fear is a stiff competitor, but can be beaten

Safe adults are no accident!

Introduction

Ready, Set, Go! Begin the Six-Step Balance System™

Talk with your physician

Before starting the Six-Step Balance System,™ talk with your doctor. If your doctor agrees that this system will be beneficial for you, set realistic goals. Then, get started! I urge you to read and sign the *Contract With Myself* on page 124. This will inspire you to make the System™ a part of your daily routine.

Fill out the Home Safety checklist

In the back of this book, you will find a useful and convenient *Home Safety Checklist*. Use this list to check "yes" or "no" as you look within your home for ways to make each room safer. Remove anything that could possibly cause anyone to fall.

Check out the pages entitled *Internet Resources*, and visit as many of these web sites as possible. To give a copy of this book to a friend, use the tear-out mailing form at the very end of the book.

To keep book open and pages laying flat, press down on binding

For easy use of this book, open and press down on the center of the book, both pages at once, so that pages will remain flat while you practice the Six-Step Balance System.™

You will be amazed at your progress. However, do not be discouraged if you do not finish every task all at once. Keep trying!

To help you minimize the fear of falling and gain the greatest benefits, this book comes with safe and easy instructions on how to perform the activities of the Six-Step Balance System.™ The more times you complete each activity, the stronger your muscles will become and the better your body will feel. **PLEASE NOTE:** Not all steps of the exercises in the book have corresponding drawings. The drawings, which were created by famous artist Jim Whiting[7] (www.jimtoons.com), will help you learn and see quickly how to perform each exercise in the correct position. As the saying goes, "A picture is worth a thousand words."

Look at the corresponding illustrations to ensure proper body position

Some of the exercises are more advanced than others; look for the "A" inside the circle and the words "advanced version" as seen to the right. You may choose to perform the alternate activities once you feel confident that you have mastered the previous skill. Each activity will help you learn to trust your every step! You will begin to trust how you are able to move your entire body. At the same time, your legs will feel stronger and you will be able to balance much better!

ADVANCED VERSION

Throughout the book you will see *Dr. Betty's Fitnotes.*[SM] Each Fitnote contains useful advice and information that can help to improve your overall health. Some contain just lighthearted observations about life.

Dr. Betty's Fitnotes[SM] offer useful advice and insight

Aim high, but always listen to your body

Aim high. Set your goals within the range of what feels comfortable for you! Always listen to your body. How you feel each day is one way you will know whether your body is getting stronger. If you are over-exercising, the aches and pains that you feel are telling you to slow down a little bit.

Set aside a specific time of day

First, set aside a specific time of day for your balance activities. Make the activities part of your routine. For instance, before brushing your teeth, your first morning cup of coffee, lunch or dinner, save just a few minutes for at least one or two of the Six-Step Balance System™ activities.

Second, stay with it. There is no substitute for practice. We all know that the more we do something, such as practicing a musical instrument, or playing golf, the better we become (well, some of us!).

A positive attitude will produce positive results

Third, keep thinking good thoughts; be optimistic. While you may not be twenty years old or an Olympic athlete, having a positive attitude is an important tool to your success. Again, it is a matter of starting slowly and practicing the activities regularly.

Practicing the activities in the Six-Step Balance System™ will give you an opportunity to improve your overall fitness and the way you live and move. It has helped literally thousands of individuals improve their balance, decrease their fear of falling and keep their bodies intact. Many have regained the ability to move more freely!

The Six-Step Balance System^{TM} has already helped thousands

A final word in this section of the book, when your loving and caring children or friends gasp and tell you, "you shouldn't do this or that," simply smile and say, "not only should I...I can!"

Yes! You can!

In my 50-plus years in the fitness arena, I have been very fortunate to share moments when people reach deep down inside and bring out their very best, overcoming their fears and living life to the fullest. And now the System is here to help you achieve the same!

To help others, whenever possible, please tell them about the Six-Step Balance System.™ Sharing the information in this book may be the greatest gift that you could ever give to family and friends!

Share the secret of the Six-Step Balance System^{TM} with friends

Wishing you the best in health and fitness,

Betty Perkins-Carpenter

Betty Perkins-Carpenter, Ph.D.

CHAPTER 1
Stretching in Bed Exercises
Balance System Step 1

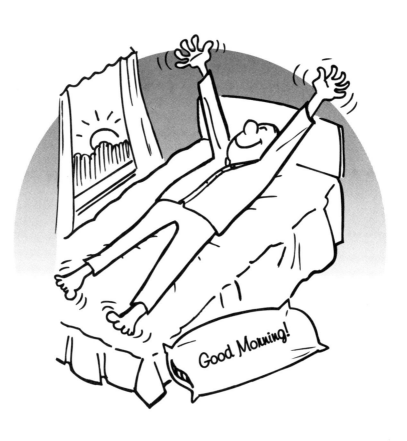

What Is Stretching and Why Is It Important?

Begin your day with a good stretch

Medical science and many years of experience have proven that stretching has great health benefits. Stretching causes muscles to warm up, making them softer and more relaxed. Warm muscles function better than cold muscles.

Stretching warms up muscles

At the same time, stretching promotes flexibility in muscles throughout the body for easier use. It helps individuals to reach, bend, push, pull and walk by reducing tension. Stretching is especially helpful for those who have arthritis or osteoporosis.

There are many benefits to stretching

While there are many reasons why people should stretch daily, some of the most well known benefits of stretching include:

- Better physical fitness overall

- Increased ability to walk safely

Stretching increases mental and physical relaxation

- Increased mental and physical relaxation

- Improved understanding of how the body moves forward, backward and sideways

- Reduced tightening of muscles and leg cramps

- Reduced soreness of muscles

- Reduced chances of injuring joints, muscles or tendons

To achieve maximum effectiveness doing the Stretching in Bed Activities:

- Turn on your favorite music. (The body is very sensitive to sound when it first wakes up.)

- Remove the pillow from behind your head.

- Lie flat on your back. For more comfort, place a pillow (or a rolled towel) under your knees.

- Perform each stretch 1 to 2 times, holding each stretch for 15 seconds. (As you improve, hold the stretch up to 30 seconds.)

- During each stretch, breathe normally. As you exhale, reach a little farther to increase each stretch. Be sure to stretch and reach as far as you can and as often as you can each day.

- Carry out every stretch in a nonstop motion. By doing so, you will place little tension on the muscle and avoid injury. (Do not jerk or bounce the stretch.)

- Never overdo it! Be sensitive to your body! Do not push yourself too hard. Stop immediately if you feel any pain!

Dr. T. Franklin Williams, former director of The National Institute on Aging, says this about Stretching In Bed: *"A short, simple program that is a great way to start your day!"* [8] You are now ready to begin the first step of the Six-Step Balance System™ with your very own stretching program. Good morning!

Turn on your favorite music

Breathe properly during your stretching exercises

Stretching in Bed Exercise #1
Wake Up Call

A stretching exercise for the whole body.

FOR STARTERS: Remove your pillow from underneath your head.

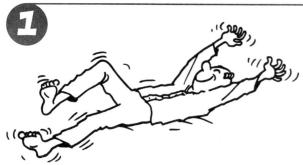

1. Stretch and reach in all directions from your fingertips to your toes!

2. Shake and wiggle, gently waking up your body.

3. Arch your back a little.

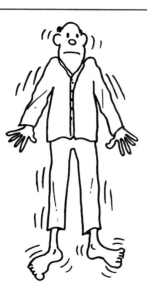

4. Now make your whole body tense from your face to your toes. Hold for 5 seconds.

5. Relax.

Stretching in Bed Exercise #2

A Little Necking

A great stretch for the neck.

FOR STARTERS: Take deep breaths by inhaling through your nose and exhaling through your mouth.

1. Turn your head slowly to the right as far as comfortable, then slowly to the left; return to center.

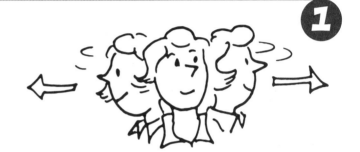

2. Next, keeping your head on the bed, make circular motions: first, in a clockwise movement, then counterclockwise.

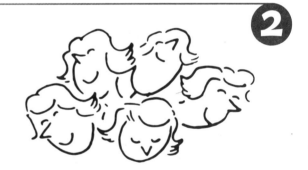

DR. BETTY'S FITNOTE™

"Stretching exercises are thought to give you more freedom of movement to do the things you need and like to do..."[9]

— National Institutes of Health

Stretching in Bed Exercise #3
High and Mighty

A stretch for the shoulders and upper back.

FOR STARTERS: Place pillow under your knees (as shown in the first illustration below).

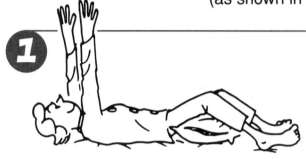

1. Stretch fingertips toward ceiling.

2. Reach with both hands. Hold for count of 3; relax.

3. Lift shoulders off bed as far as you can; lower shoulders, pushing gently into the bed; relax.

4. Reach toward the ceiling with right hand only; relax. Then, repeat with left hand.

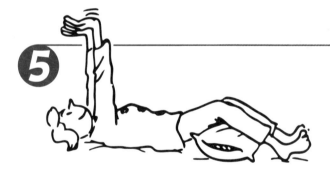

5. Now, with palms flat, stretch both hands toward ceiling; hold and relax.

6. Stretch fingertips toward feet, point your toes down; hold, relax.

7. Finally, keeping arms straight with palms down, move both hands and arms as far right across the bed as possible.

8. Stretch, relax. Repeat to left side.

Elbow Magic

Another stretch for the shoulders and upper back.

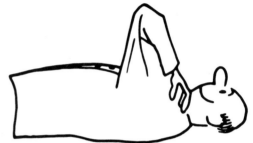

1. Place fingertips on your shoulders, and raise elbows pointing to the ceiling.

2. Then, lower elbows to bed while keeping fingertips on shoulders.

3. Lift elbows again, but this time touch your elbows together in front of you, or as close as you can, without straining.

4. Then, lower elbows to bed.

5. Now, keeping fingers on your shoulders, make 5 large circles clockwise with both elbows, then repeat 5 times counterclockwise.

Stretching in Bed Exercise #5
Rock 'N' Roll

A stretch for the waist, hips and thighs.

 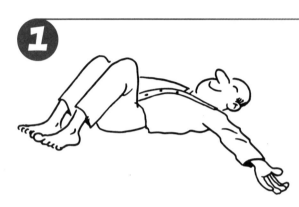

1. Place arms out to your sides (slightly below shoulder level), bend your knees.

2. With head still and shoulders flat on bed, roll onto your right hip as far as possible, keeping your knees and feet together.

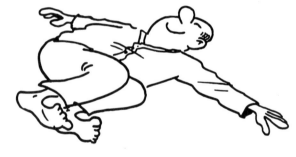

3. Return to center and roll to the left side.

4. Alternate right and left, 2 to 4 times.

Stretching in Bed Exercise #6

It's All in the Wrists

A stretch for the hands, fingers and shoulders.

1. Stretch your arms straight up in the air, finger-tips pointing at the ceiling.

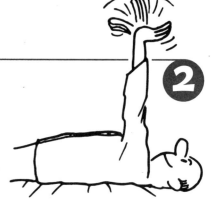

2. Flex your wrists, so that you're waving your hands up and down.

3. Keep waving as you move your arms out to the sides and down to the bed. Continue waving as you return your arms to the starting position.

4. Now, flex hands at the wrists, moving your fingertips left to right, like windshield wipers.

5. Rotate your wrists, tracing circles with your fingertips on the ceiling, clockwise, then counterclockwise.

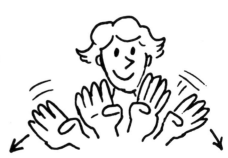

Finger Fun

A stretch for the hands and fingers.

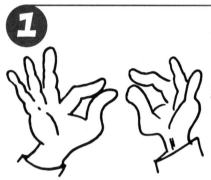

1. Touch your index fingers to the thumbs of the same hand; then open them wide and stretch.

2. Continue by touching the other fingers to your thumbs with a stretch in between.

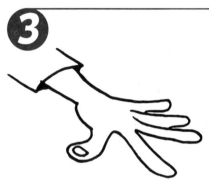

3. Then, with both hands on the bed, palms down, press each finger into the bed one at a time.

4. Raise your hands and "shake out" fingers and wrists.

5. Relax.

Stretching in Bed Exercise #8

I Love Me

A stretch for the lower back.

1. With both knees comfortably bent and feet flat, pull right thigh gently toward chest by placing hands under knees.

2. Now, hug yourself; release and return to starting position.

3. Repeat with left knee; relax.

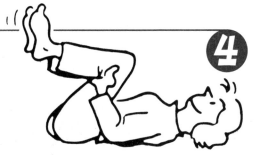

4. Next, draw both knees toward chest and hold for 10 seconds; relax.

5. Return to starting position.

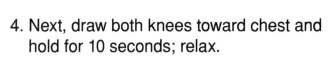

6. Now, slightly arch back; relax.

7. Then, pull in stomach and flatten your back against the bed.

8. Hold for a slow count of 3 and relax.

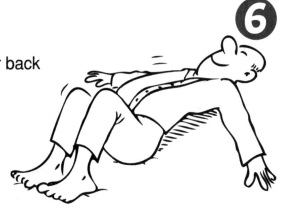

Stretching in Bed Exercise #9
Kick Up Your Heels

A stretch for the hips and back of legs.

1. With knees bent, bring left knee toward your chest, as far as comfortable.

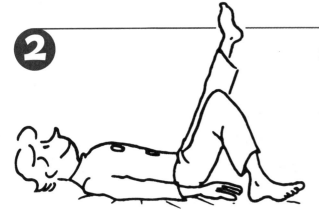

2

2. Straighten left leg up toward ceiling as far as you are able.

3. Then, bend knee and lower foot to bed.

4. Repeat with right leg.

DR. BETTY'S
FITNOTE™

"The point of stretching isn't so you can scratch your ears with your feet. It's so you can climb in and out of the car with ease, slip into your coat and pick-up change from the sidewalk."

– Bob Anderson, Author of *Stretching*, www.stretching.com

Stretching in Bed Exercise #10
Windshield Wipers

A stretch for the ankles.

1. Point your toes down as far as your can; then turn each foot in so toes face each other.

2. Next, turn them out so heels face each other. Now, pretend your feet are windshield wipers.

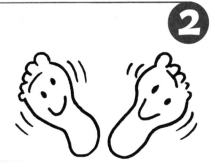

3. Turn both feet together, first to the right...

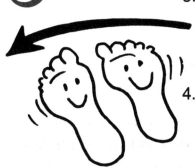

4. Then, turn them to the left. (You may also complete circles clockwise and counterclockwise.)

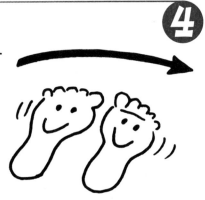

Stretching in Bed Exercise #11
Fancy Footwork

Stretch those toes and feet.

①

1. Curl your toes down as far as you can, then spread them wide open.

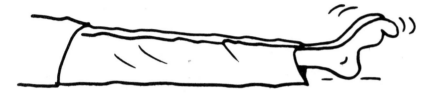

②

2. Jiggle and wiggle your toes every which way.

3. Repeat, as often as it feels good.

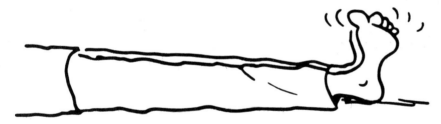

Stretching in Bed Exercise #12
There and Back Again

A stretch for the hips.

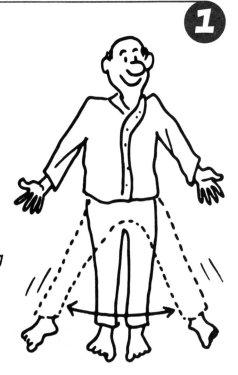

1. With your legs straight, slowly **SLIDE** your heels (do not lift your legs) as far apart as possible.

2. Keep toes pointed upward.

3. Keeping heels on the bed, slide your legs back together.

4. Repeat 3 times.

NOTE: The illustration here represents a top-down view. When performing this stretching exercise, imagine you're looking down on yourself in bed to gain perspective of correct body position. Palms facing up or down is a matter of choice.

Rise to the Occasion

Stretch that back.

1. Lie face down, with your palms down, arms bent at elbows, and forearms on the bed.

2. Slowly lift upper body and hold for 10 seconds.

3. Lower your chest and head to bed; relax.

4. Repeat 3 times. Relax between each stretch for 3 to 5 seconds.

DR. BETTY'S FITNOTE™

"Too many people confine their exercise to jumping to conclusions, running up bills, stretching the truth, bending over backward, lying down on the job, sidestepping responsibility and pushing their luck." — Author unknown

Stretching in Bed Exercise #14
Victory Stretch

A stretch for the upper body, waist and lower back.

1. Sit with legs apart, feet on the floor, arms and hands at your side, looking straight ahead, extend your right arm out in front of you.

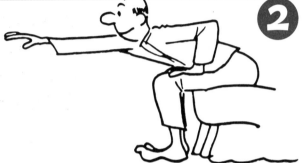

2. Place left hand on top of your left thigh. Bend over at the waist and reach for the wall in front of you with your right arm.

3. Return to starting position.

4. Alternate sides and repeat 5 times.

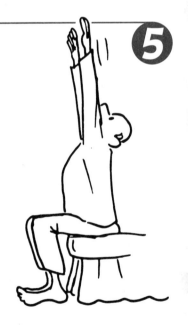

5. Now, stretch with both arms up toward the ceiling, looking up just a little bit; lower arms to sides; relax.

6. Now, bend to the right, then left, as though you are swaying in the wind; relax.

CHAPTER 2
Balance Exercises
Balance System Step 2

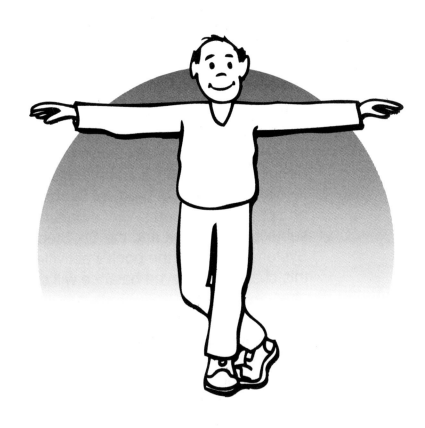

What Is Balance and Why Is It Important?

How is the word "balance" defined?

We have all heard the word "balance" used in many situations to describe many different things. In the Six-Step Balance System,™ I define balance as "the ability of the body to keep its center of gravity in order to avoid a fall."

For a clinical definition, MedicineNet.com[11] defines balance as "A biological system that enables us to know where our bodies are in the environment and to maintain a desired position."

Keeping one's balance is a complex process. It involves the use of many of the body's mental and physical attributes. Since balance is the main subject of this book and the Six-Step Balance System,™ most of the book's activities are in this chapter. Improved balance will decrease the chances of a fall.

The brain feeds a constant flow of information to the body

To balance safely, one must rely on a constant flow of information to and from the brain about how the body is positioned. Nerves, muscles, bones and overall body movement receive instructions from the brain telling the body how to perform the changes needed to maintain balance.

Information about body position comes from three sources:

1. The eyes, which give visual information about the body's position in relation to its surroundings

2. Sensory nerves in the skin, muscles and joints (called proprioceptors), which provide information about the position and movement of the different parts of the body

3. Vestibular system (part of the inner-ear), an extremely important source of sensory information that the brain needs to assist in controlling balance

These organized and easy-to-follow activities will take you on a comfortable journey from the fun and simple "getting started" balance movements to the fun and "more advanced" balance movements.

While many activities of the Six-Step Balance System™ do not require that you buy any special equipment, you will need to use simple "props."

For example, you will need a chair, ball, pillow and a balance beam. (More about making your own floor balance beam in **Recommendation #2** on page 61).

Body position comes from three sources

Balance activities DO NOT require any expensive equipment

Balance Exercise #1

Find Your Balance Point

Before you try any of the Balance Exercises, familiarize yourself with your "balance point" and a few simple warm-up activities. You will find that the majority of Balance Exercises ask you to begin by finding this important reference point.

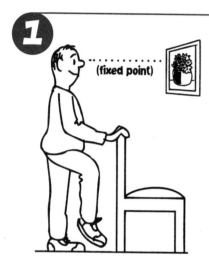

(fixed point)

1

NOTE! For some, it may be uncomfortable at first to raise a foot off the floor. Continue practicing by holding on to the back of a chair until you feel safe and confident.

Because we are all unique, we each have our own balance point or center of gravity. By this I mean the position in which, when you are balancing, your weight is evenly distributed and you feel comfortable and safe.

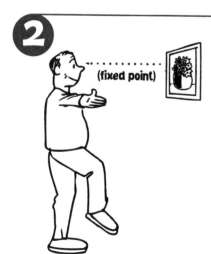

(fixed point)

2

As seen in the illustrations 1 and 2 to the left, you may or may not need a chair for stability during the process of staring at a fixed point as you lift one foot slightly off the floor. A fixed point can be a spot on the wall, a picture or anywhere that you "feel" in balance.

There are also several variations *continued on the next page*. Practice the position of your choice and let it become second nature to you as you continue with the rest of the Balance Exercises.

Balance Exercise #1

Find Your Balance Point

(continued from previous page)

As you can see from the illustrations, there are several positions in which you may be most comfortable balancing. If you at anytime feel uneasy, try the positions below with both feet shoulder-width apart. Try doing so with:

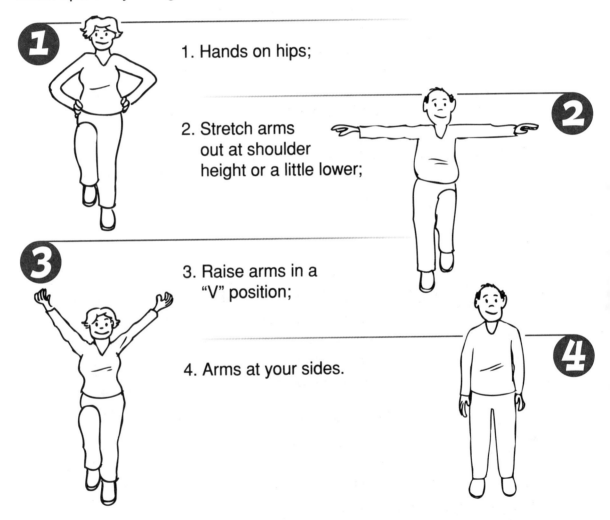

1. Hands on hips;

2. Stretch arms out at shoulder height or a little lower;

3. Raise arms in a "V" position;

4. Arms at your sides.

Balance Exercise #2

Shake It Up & Stretch

Gets your whole body feeling loose and relaxed.

FOR STARTERS: Stand tall with your feet comfortably apart and arms loosely at your sides.

1. Stretch your arms up over your head, then stretch them out to the sides; next, stretch your fingertips down toward the floor.

2. Now, RELAX. Try to feel an overall "looseness," as if your arms and whole body were "cooked spaghetti." Allow everything to hang loose – your face, eyes and neck, down to your toes.

3. Next, shake your loose right arm. Shake your loose left arm.

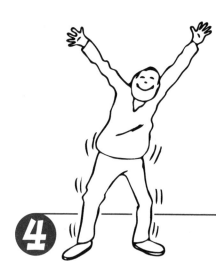

4. Shake your loose right leg, then your loose left leg.

5. Now, wiggle your "okole" (Hawaiian for buttocks).

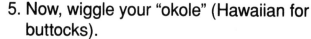

6. Keep moving your arms, legs and okole until you feel completely loose and relaxed.

Balance Exercise #3

Elevator Going Up & Down

Do this activity every day to increase leg strength.

FOR STARTERS: Sit in a stationary chair. Feet should be a comfortable distance apart and arms should be at your sides with hands resting on your knees or thighs, whichever is best for you.

Make believe you are on an elevator going up one floor at a time and stopping (holding your position) for a few seconds at each floor. Let's use a four-story building.

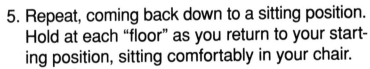

1. Stand up a little and hold (first floor).

2. Stand up a little higher and hold (second floor).

3. Stand up higher still and hold (third floor).

4. Now stand up tall as the elevator reaches the top (fourth floor).

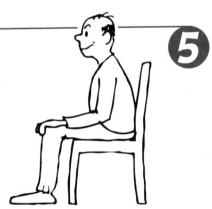

5. Repeat, coming back down to a sitting position. Hold at each "floor" as you return to your starting position, sitting comfortably in your chair.

Balance Exercise #4

Barefoot in the Park

Great exercise for the muscles in your feet.

FOR STARTERS: Lie flat on the floor, in bed, or sit tall in a chair.

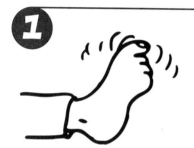

1. Curl and tense your toes as tightly as you can. Hold for a *slow* count of 3, then uncurl and relax.

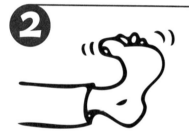

2. Next, wiggle your toes and relax.

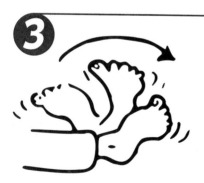

3. Now, "flutter" your feet one at a time (like you would your eyelashes).

4. Relax and "shake out" your feet.

REPETITIONS: 8 times, each foot.

(continued on next page)

Balance Exercise #4
Barefoot in the Park

(continued from previous page)

Here are a few warm-up activities for your feet, that, incidentally, also help prevent sprained ankles.

- Spread your toes wide within your shoes and then curl them under. If you can't do this, *BUY NEW SHOES*! Spreading toes wide helps you to stabilize yourself if and when you lose your balance.

- Play games with your toes. With bare feet, try to pick up marbles and move them from one spot to another.

- Place a sock on the floor, then try and pick it up with your toes.

- Massage your feet and each toe, using your thumbs.

- Lift toes up off the floor, then lower. Then lift heels up, then lower.

Now, let's join the Army:

- Lift right heel up, then down. Lift left heel up, then down. Now very quickly, Right! Left! Right! Left! 10 times, as if you were in the Army.

Buy new shoes if you can't spread your toes

Recommendation #1
Athletic Footwear

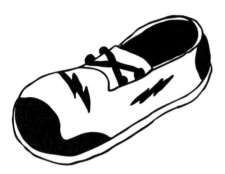

I believe that it is extremely important for you to have the proper footwear when performing the Six-Step Balance System.™ My friends at The American Academy of Orthopedic Surgeons offer these tips when buying shoes:[12]

Try on new shoes at the end of the day. Your feet normally swell and become larger after standing or sitting during the day. There should be a firm grip of the shoe to your heel. Your heel should not slip as you walk. Try on both left and right shoes.

Fit new shoes to your largest foot. Most people have one foot larger than the other. There should be 1/2-inch space from the end of your longest toe to the front of the shoe. Walk around the store in the shoes to make sure they fit well and feel comfortable. Sizes vary among shoe brands and styles.

Judge a shoe by how it fits on your foot, not by the marked size. When the shoe is on your foot, you should be able to wiggle all of your toes freely. Curl your toes under and then spread them wide. If the shoes feel too tight and you cannot spread your toes wide, don't buy them! There is no such thing as a "break-in period." Wearing tightly fitted shoes or loosely fitted shoes could mean the difference between regaining your balance and avoiding a fall. Also, if your feet hurt, you will not want to engage in any activities!

If you have any specific foot problem, seek help from a podiatrist. Shop around for proper care and help for your feet. Your feet are the only two that you have; take care of them with the best care available. You will be glad you did!

Balance Exercise #5

Tootsies Roll

Find a rolling pin or can of soup for this exercise.

FOR STARTERS: Stand (preferably) or sit tall, with bare feet. If you do this exercise while standing, please be sure to hold on to the back of a straight chair or counter for balance and safety.

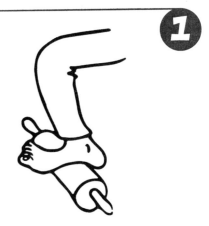

1. Place a rolling pin on the floor and put the arch of your foot on it.

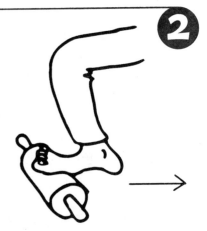

2. Now, slowly roll your foot backward over the pin (to the tips of your toes). Then roll your foot forward all the way to your heel. Increase pressure gradually, especially under the arch.

3. Repeat the rolling movements with your other foot. (Always exercise both feet, even if you think only one foot needs it.)

REPETITIONS: 2 to 3 times with each foot.

Balance Exercise #6

One for the Books

You'll need a phone book or thick novel for this one.

FOR STARTERS: Stand tall, with feet slightly apart on the floor (Important: Keep good posture – back straight, shoulders back). As an alternative, try this exercise sitting down.

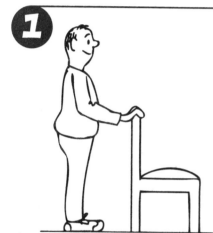

1

1. Hold on to the back of a straight chair and slowly raise both heels until your weight is on the balls of your feet. Hold for a *slow* count of 3.

2. Lower and relax.

3. Repeat 5 to 10 times.

(continued on next page)

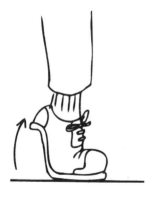

DR. BETTY'S FITNOTE™

"Foot and ankle characteristics, particularly tactile sensitivity, ankle flexibility and toe strength are important determinants of balance and functional ability in older people." [13]

– Hylton B. Menz

Balance Exercise #6

One for the Books

(continued from previous page)

4. Now, position a book on the floor so that the binding is facing you.

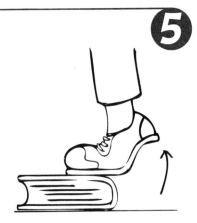

5. Hold on to the back of a straight chair and with the front half of your feet, step up onto the book one foot at a time. Slowly raise both heels until your weight is on the balls of your feet.

6. Hold for a *slow* count of 3. Lower and relax.

7. Repeat 5 to 10 times.

REPETITIONS: Repeat entire exercise 1 to 3 times.

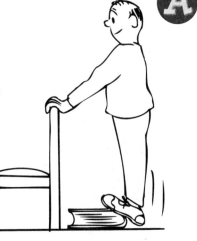

ADVANCED VERSION

For an even more advanced version, go back to the phone book and this time when you raise and lower your heels, stop every 2 inches, holding each position for a *slow* count of 3.

Balance Exercise #7

First Steps

This exercise is very important to do well.

FOR STARTERS: Stand tall with feet slightly apart. Place both hands on the back of a stationary chair in front of you.

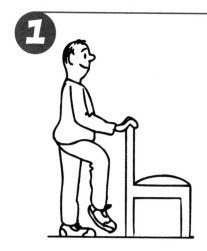

1. Holding onto the chair, raise your right knee so your foot is a few inches off the floor (a little higher once you've mastered the movements). Allow your right leg, from knee to foot, to hang loose. Be careful not to tuck your foot under your thigh!

2. Hold this position for a *slow* count of 3. Return right leg to starting position and relax.

3. Perform the activity with your left leg. Now, repeat once with right leg, then with left leg.

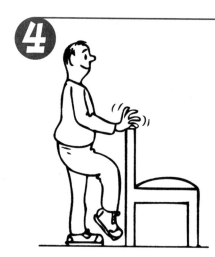

4. Now, "play the piano" by rippling your fingertips on the back of the chair. (By this I mean practice how it feels to balance without the complete support of the chair.)

5. While "playing piano," repeat lifting your right knee and then your left knee (steps 1, 2 & 3 above) just high enough to sense how it might feel to let go of the chair completely.

(continued on next page)

Balance Exercise #7
First Steps

(continued from previous page)

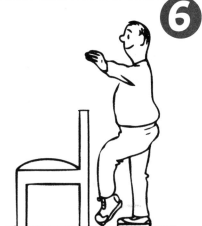

6. Now, raise your right knee so that your foot is a few inches off the floor. Slowly, and relaxed, let go of the chair and gently raise your arms, little by little, until you find your balance point.

7. Hold this position as long as you can. (At first, it might be just a fraction of a second, but gradually you will be able to hold your position for longer intervals.)

8. Return your hands to the chair and lower your right leg. RELAX.

9. Repeat with your left leg.

Remember to maintain your posture (straight back).

REPETITIONS: 4 to 5 times.

DR. BETTY'S FITNOTE™

REMEMBER: Your "Balance Point" refers to the position in which, when you are balancing, your weight is evenly positioned and you feel comfortable, safe and secure.

Balance Exercise #8
Chorus Line

Concentrate and focus for this one.

FOR STARTERS: Stand tall, feet together and arms at your chosen balance point.

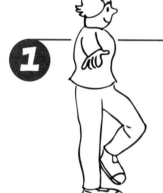

1. Lift your left knee so that your foot is just off the floor.

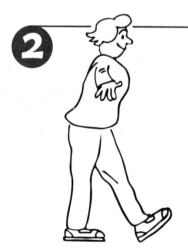

2. Straighten your left leg out in front of you, but don't touch the floor.

3. Return to bent-knee position and lower left foot to the floor. *(Refer to illustration #1)*

4. Relax and repeat activity using your right leg.

REPETITIONS: 3 times.

(continued on next page)

Balance Exercise #8
Chorus Line

(continued from previous page)

(continued from previous page)

ADVANCED VERSION

1. When your leg is straightened, point your toes and really S-T-R-E-T-C-H.

2. Hold the stretch for a *slow* count of 3. **FEEL** those leg muscles work!

3. Gently "push" your heel forward, toward the floor. Hold for a *slow* count of 3.

4. Flex your ankle to bring your toes up toward your body, then down, away from your body.

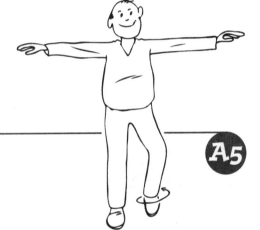

5. Gently, with the ankle very loose and relaxed, rotate your ankle clockwise and then counterclockwise.

REPETITIONS: Do as many as you are comfortable doing.

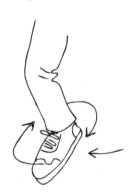

DR. BETTY'S FITNOTE™

You may get cramps from stretching. If you do, drink lots of water, as you could be dehydrated. You may also choose to do fewer repetitions.

Balance Exercise #9

Heel-To-Toe

A terrific exercise to strengthen the ankles.

FOR STARTERS: Stand tall, feet slightly apart and arms at balance point.

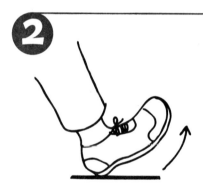

1. Relax and then raise your left leg straight out in front of you, with your foot just off the floor.

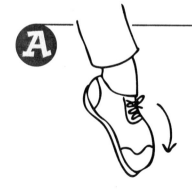

2. Now, touch your heel to the floor, then touch your toes to the floor. Repeat heel-to-toe, touching 4 times.

3. Lower left leg and relax.

4. Repeat the activity with your right leg.

REPETITIONS: 2 or 3 times, with both legs.

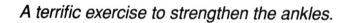

ADVANCED VERSION

Do not allow heel or toe to touch floor. Flex your ankle and do Heel-To-Toe "in the air." It takes time to build your self-confidence. Be delighted with every improvement, because you know it means you're reducing the risk of a fall!

Balance Exercise #10

Swing Time

Be sure to rest from time to time during workouts.

FOR STARTERS: Stand tall, feet slightly apart and arms at your balance point.

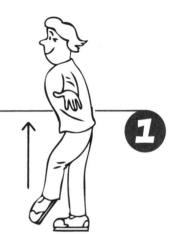

1. Lift your left knee so that your foot is comfortably off the floor.

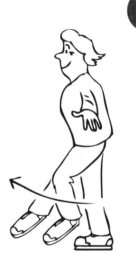

2. Gently swing your lower leg from the knee to the foot, forward and backward, like a pendulum, 5 times.

3. Lower your leg and relax.

4. Repeat the activity with your right leg.

REPETITIONS: Alternating your left and right legs, repeat steps 1 to 3 as many times as you wish.

DR. BETTY'S FITNOTE™

"A bird doesn't sing because it has an answer, it sings because it has a song."

– Maya Angelou, American writer (1928-)

Balance Exercise #11

A Real Swinger

Now you're really starting to improve your balance.

FOR STARTERS: Stand tall, feet slightly apart, arms at your balance point.

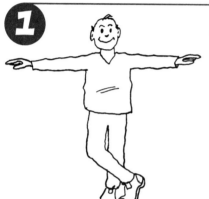

1. Bend your right knee and cross your right foot in front of and to the outside of your left foot, touching your right toes to the floor. Now you are a swinger.

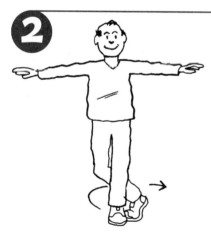

2. With knee still bent, gently swing your right leg from the front position to behind your left leg, touching your right toes to the floor.

3. Return to starting position; relax, and repeat activity using your left leg.

REPETITIONS: 4 times with right and left leg. You may prefer alternating. Your choice!

(continued on next page)

Balance Exercise #11

A Real Swinger

(continued from previous page)

ADVANCED VERSION

Practice being "A Real Swinger" without touching your toes to the floor. This may take some time to master!

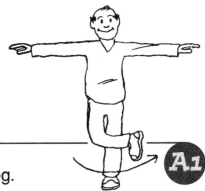

1. Gently swing your right leg in front of your left leg.

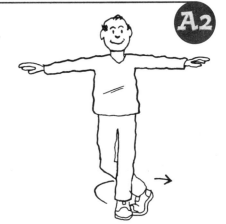

2. Gently swing your right leg behind your left leg.

3. Gently swing right leg out to the side, then return.

4. Gently swing your right leg in front, out to the side, then behind your left leg.

5. Return to starting position, relax and repeat activity using your left leg.

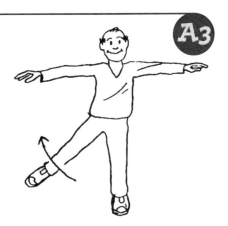

Balance Exercise #12
Flamingo Dance

Be sure to breathe normally during exercises.

FOR STARTERS: Stand tall, feet slightly apart and arms at balance point.

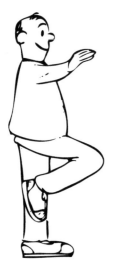

1. Raise your left knee and place your left foot on the inside of your right calf. Hold for a *slow* count of 3.

2. Now, slowly SLIDE your left foot down your right calf to the floor.

3. Relax, then repeat activity using your right foot.

REPETITIONS: Alternate legs 3 to 4 times.

ADVANCED VERSION

You can greatly increase the difficulty of Flamingo Dance by lifting your foot higher and resting it on the inside of the knee.

Then, slowly slide your foot down to the calf, stop and hold for a *slow* count of 3; lower to ankle and hold for a *slow* count of 3; then back to the floor. Repeat with other foot. You can also move your foot up and down your leg as if you were "scratching a mosquito bite."

Balance Exercise #13

Balance Ballet

Ladies, remember when you were a ballerina?

FOR STARTERS: Stand tall, feet slightly apart and arms at balance point.

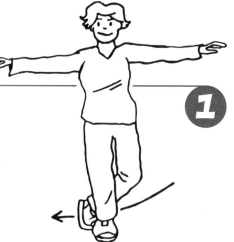

1. Bend your left knee and bring your left leg behind your right leg, so that the left leg is resting low on the right calf, toes on the floor.

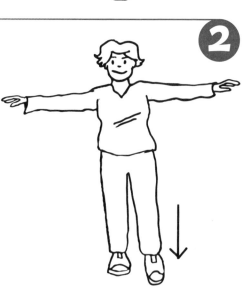

2. Return your left leg back to the starting position and stretch it out in front of you, toes pointed down, just above the floor.

3. Return to the starting position and relax.

4. Repeat the activity using your right leg.

REPETITIONS: 2 to 3 times.

(continued on next page)

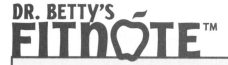

DR. BETTY'S
FITNOTE™

> **"Success is a marathon, not a sprint."**
> **– Unknown**

Balance Exercise #13
Balance Ballet

(continued from previous page)

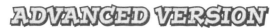

Challenge yourself! Repeat steps 1 and 2 a total of 4 times without touching the floor.

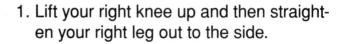

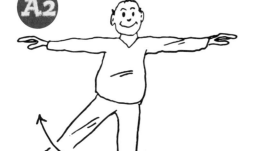

1. Lift your right knee up and then straighten your right leg out to the side.

2. Gently swing your leg sideways out and in, then out and in again.

3. Repeat with left leg.

   REPETITIONS: 1 to 2 times

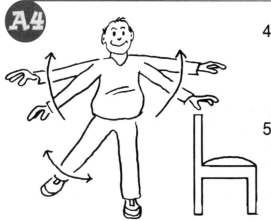

4. With a chair beside you, place your left hand on top of the chair, then lift both arms up and at the same time lift your right leg up and out to the side.

5. Lower your arms and right leg and repeat using left leg. (Turn around so that your right hand is on top of the chair).

   REPETITIONS: 2 to 3 times

Balance Exercise #14

Raise Your Hand

This is also a mental-physical exercise.

FOR STARTERS: Stand tall, feet slightly apart and arms at balance point.

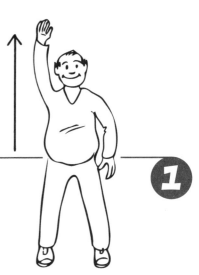

1. Stretch your right arm over your head as far as is comfortable for you.

2. With your right arm still extended, raise your left knee as high as you comfortably can.

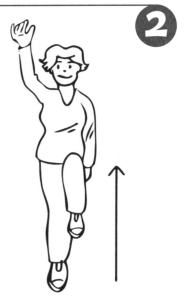

3. Lower your right arm and left leg and relax.

4. Repeat using the left arm and right leg.

REPETITIONS: Repeat 2 to 3 times.

(continued on next page)

DR. BETTY'S FITNOTE™

A doctor complained to his patient, "That check you gave me for my doctor bill came back." The patient replied, "Yep! And so did my arthritis."

— Golden Horizons, Inc.

Raise Your Hand

(continued from previous page)

ADVANCED VERSION

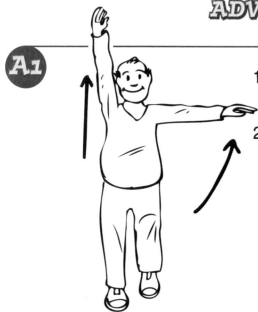

A1

1. Raise your right arm over your head and, at the same time, raise your left knee.

2. Holding that position, lower right arm and raise left arm until both arms are at shoulder level.

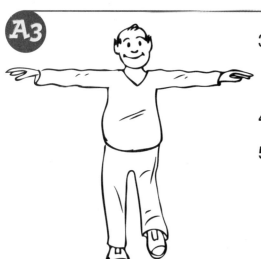

A3

3. Now, straighten left leg out to the front without touching the floor; hold for *slow* count of 3, bend knee, lower leg and relax.

4. Lower arms and relax.

5. Repeat using the left arm and right leg.

REPETITIONS: As many as you enjoy!

Recommendation #2

Constructing a floor balance beam

Some of the following Balance activities will require you to use a "floor balance beam" that you can easily make yourself. Since we don't have regulation beams in our homes, we have to be creative and make our own! Simply lay down strips of masking tape about 8′ long on a rug or on the floor. Depending on the width of your tape, you will put down 2 to 4 strips, side by side, so that your "beam" is 4″ wide.

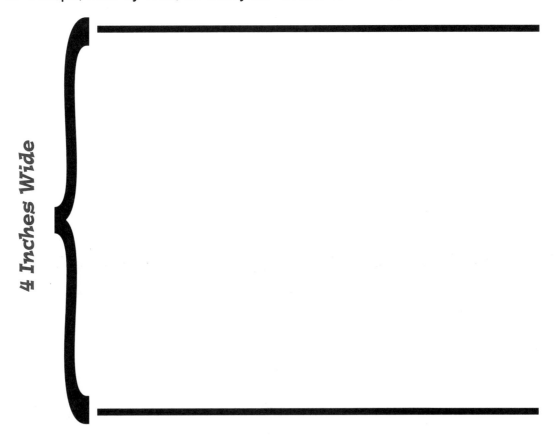

4 Inches Wide

If you have a straight line in the pattern of your rug, or squares (tiles) on the floor, you may have a "ready made" balance beam. (Remember to place your "beam" in an area you use frequently. The more you practice, the safer you'll be!)

Balance Exercise #15
Tightrope Walker

This exercise extends for the next 3 pages.

FOR STARTERS: Stand comfortably in front of your masking tape "balance beam."

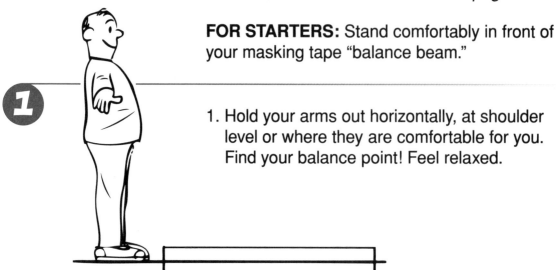

1. Hold your arms out horizontally, at shoulder level or where they are comfortable for you. Find your balance point! Feel relaxed.

START   FINISH

2. Stepping very slowly (without running down the "beam"), place one foot in front of the other on the beam. It doesn't matter which foot you start with, but do try to space your feet about four (4) inches apart (between the heel of the leading foot and the toe of the trailing foot) and feel in good balance. You should try to walk normally, but you might want to experiment turning your toes out and your heels in a bit for better balance. Be sure to "feel" your balance point each time before going on.

(continued on next page)

Tightrope Walker

(continued from previous page)

③

3. Continue walking along the beam. Your eyes should focus on the end of the beam (3 or 4 feet in front of you, or on a target straight ahead at eye level). Do not look down at your feet, it will cause you to move out of balance.

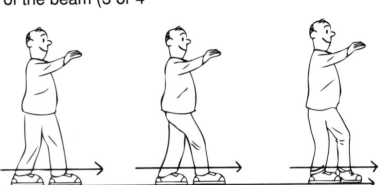

4. Walk to the end of the beam slowly, staying on the parallel taped lines. Your arms will automatically move freely, helping you to maintain your balance with each step. If you're barefoot, in socks or stockings, FEEL the tape with your toes. Sensory perception in our feet is very important to balance.

5. When you reach the end, lower your arms and relax. Now, turn around and walk the beam back. (As you turn, focus your eyes straight ahead.) Be sure to maintain good posture.

REPETITIONS: Do at least once or twice daily! If your fear of falling is great, you may wish to start with the variations on the next page.

(continued on next page)

Balance Exercise #15

Tightrope Walker

(continued from previous page)

1. Place your right foot on the beam and your left foot off the beam and walk normally to the end. Turn and come back with your left foot on the beam and your right foot off.

2. Stand with both feet on the beam and move your right foot forward. Bring your left foot forward to meet your right foot; step forward, close, repeat. Then, starting with your left foot, repeat the above.

3. Stand on beam facing sideways and slowly slide your right foot to the right and bring your left foot to meet right foot. Continue sliding sideways to the end of the beam. Return sliding sideways to the left, starting with the left foot.

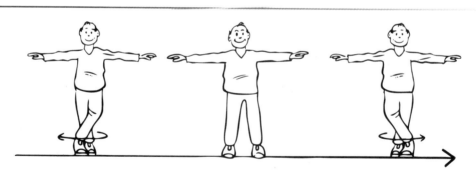

ADVANCED VERSION

For fun, walk forward and backward. Or, try "crossovers." Cross your left foot over your right, going to the right on the "beam." Then, cross right over left on your return trip.

Balance Exercise #16

Pedaler's Poise

This will bring back memories of riding your bicycle.

FOR STARTERS: Stand tall, feet slightly apart and arms at your balance point.

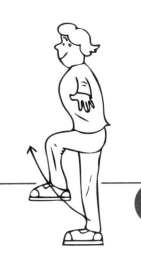

1. Raise your right knee, putting your foot on a make-believe bicycle pedal, just off the floor.

2. Start to "pedal" by moving your right foot in a downward, circular path brushing the floor with your toes. (Remember to point your toes down, just as you would on a real bike pedal. This will also increase your ankle flexibility!)

3. Return your right foot to the floor and relax.

4. Repeat the activity using your left leg.

REPETITIONS: 3 rotations each leg.

ADVANCED VERSION

Don't touch the floor with your toes! Then, increase the degree of difficulty by lifting your knee higher and higher off the floor, making larger circles with your "pedaling" motion. Also go in reverse! Pedal backward!

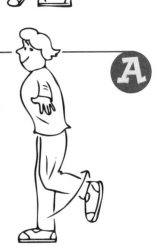

(continued on next page)

Balance Exercise #16
Pedaler's Poise

(continued from previous page)

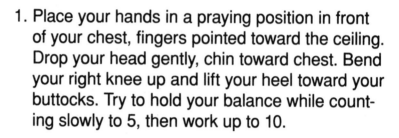 Variations

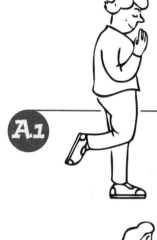

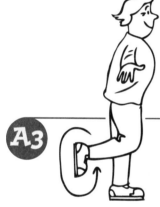

1. Place your hands in a praying position in front of your chest, fingers pointed toward the ceiling. Drop your head gently, chin toward chest. Bend your right knee up and lift your heel toward your buttocks. Try to hold your balance while counting slowly to 5, then work up to 10.

2. Bend your right knee down and gently place the toes of your right foot on the floor behind you.

3. Lift your right heel up toward your buttocks and move your toes in a small, slow, gentle circle, first clockwise and then counterclockwise.

4. Lower foot to floor and repeat with left leg. Relax.

5. Lift your right leg out to the side and complete 2 small circles clockwise.

6. Lower leg and relax.

7. Repeat using your left leg.

REPETITIONS: 1 to 2 times

Balance Exercise #17

You're In The Army Now

...or Air Force, Marines, Navy or Coast Guard

FOR STARTERS: Stand tall, with your feet slightly apart.

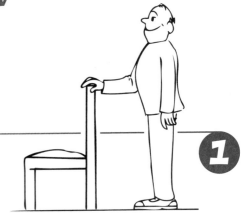

1. With hand resting on a stationary chair in front of you, stand at attention. Ten-hut, soldier, it's march time!

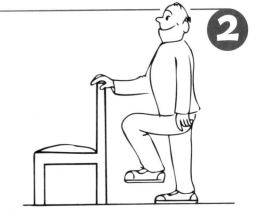

2. Holding onto the back of the chair for support, alternate lifting your right knee, then your left. March in place for a count of 1 - 2, 1 - 2 - 3, 1 - 2, 1 - 2 - 3, etc. (Cadence counting makes it more fun.)

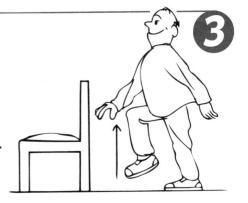

3. Still marching in place as above, slowly let go of the chair. Swing your arms to the rhythm of your feet.

REPETITIONS: 30 seconds to 1 minute or more; this gradually increases your endurance.

(continued on next page)

Balance Exercise #17

You're In The Army Now

(continued from previous page)

ADVANCED VERSION

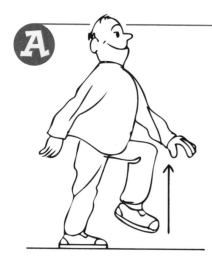

Ⓐ

Move away from the chair. Really swing those arms! March as if you were in the army; and then, as you lift your left arm and right leg – stop – and hold them both momentarily. Then, lower your arm and leg and march again.

Repeat by raising right arm and left leg. (As you gently swing your arms, you are maintaining your shoulder flexibility and endurance.)

DR. BETTY'S FITNOTE™

"nobody gets to live life backward. Look ahead – that's where your future lies."

– Ann Landers, Advice Columnist (1918-2002)

Tap Dance

Tap dancing classes — Remember?

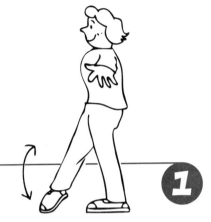

FOR STARTERS: Stand tall with your feet slightly apart and arms at your balance point.

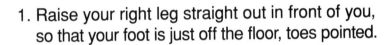

1. Raise your right leg straight out in front of you, so that your foot is just off the floor, toes pointed.

2. Move your leg up and down 3 times, tapping the floor with your toes each time.

3. Return to starting position; repeat with left leg.

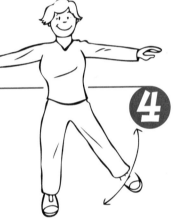

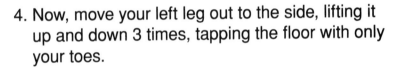

4. Now, move your left leg out to the side, lifting it up and down 3 times, tapping the floor with only your toes.

5. Repeat using your right leg.

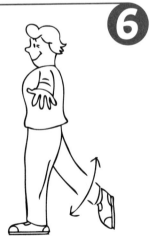

6. Next, move your right leg around behind you and tap your toes 3 times.

7. Return to starting position and relax; repeat activity using your left leg.

REPETITIONS: 2 times.

ADVANCED VERSION

To increase the difficulty, don't touch the floor while "tapping."

Balance Exercise #19

Balancing Act

This exercise reduces the fear of falling forward.

FOR STARTERS: Rest your hands on the back of a chair as lightly as possible.

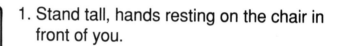

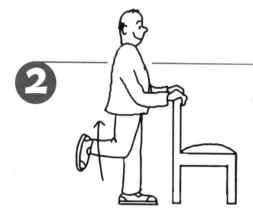

1. Stand tall, hands resting on the chair in front of you.

2. Bend your right leg at the knee so that your foot is behind you.

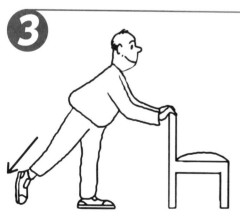

3. Lean slightly forward toward the chair. Straighten your right leg out behind you to a comfortable position and gently point your toes. Then bend your knee. Return to starting position and relax.

4. Repeat the activity with your left leg. (Be sure you have become comfortable with steps 1 - 3 before going on to next page!)

Balance Exercise #19

Balancing Act

(continued from previous page)

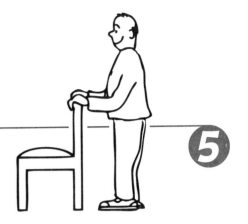

5. Stand tall, hands resting on the chair in front of you.

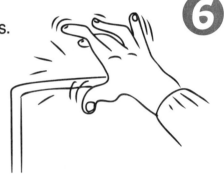

6. "Play the piano" on the chair with your fingertips.

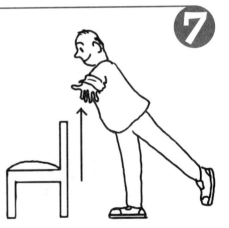

7. Now, slowly raise your arms to your balance point. Extend your left leg out behind you as you lean toward the chair. Hold for a *slow* count of 3.

8. Repeat using your right leg.

9. Now, move your feet a little farther away from the chair and repeat all of the steps.

REPETITIONS: 1 to 2 times.

Tipsy: Sideward Movement

Great exercise for whittling your waist, too.

FOR STARTERS: Sit tall in an armless chair. (If you do not have an armless chair, place your arms on the outside of the arms of your chair.)

1. Arms out to side at shoulder height.

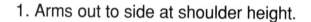

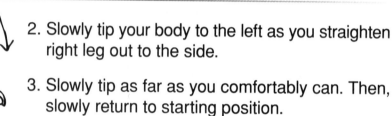

2. Slowly tip your body to the left as you straighten right leg out to the side.

3. Slowly tip as far as you comfortably can. Then, slowly return to starting position.

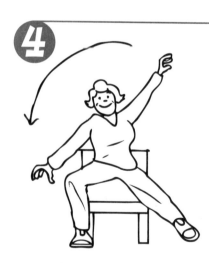

4. Repeat to right side lifting and straightening left leg.

REPETITIONS: 3 to 4 times.

For fun, and between repetitions, practice "Upsa-Daisy." Stand up, sit down, stand up, turn around and sit down.

Balance Exercise #21

Steady As She Goes

This exercise reduces the fear of falling sideways.

FOR STARTERS: Stand tall, feet slightly apart, with your left hand resting on a stationary chair beside you.

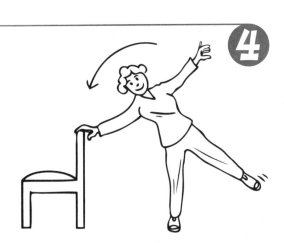

1. With left hand on the chair, raise your right leg out to the side and your right arm to a comfortable balance point.

2. Hold the position for a *slow* count of 5. **Steady as she goes!**

3. Return to starting position and relax.

4. Repeat the activity with your right hand on chair and using your left leg and left arm.

REPETITIONS: 3 times.

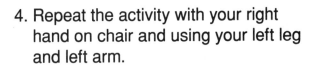

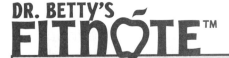

DR. BETTY'S
FITNOTE™

> **"Courage is being scared to death, but saddling up anyway."** – John Wayne, American actor (1907-1979)

Balance Exercise #22

Hip Hip Hooray!

Hip Hip Hooray is a very advanced activity!

FOR STARTERS: (Be sure you are experienced and feel safe and secure with all the other balance activities before proceeding.) The first time you try these movements, you may wish to use a chair that has been placed against a wall so it cannot move. Stand tall, feet slightly apart, arms at your balance point.

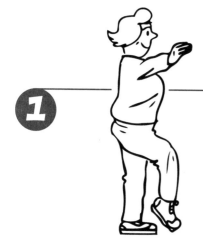

1

1. Lift your right knee so your foot is just off the floor.

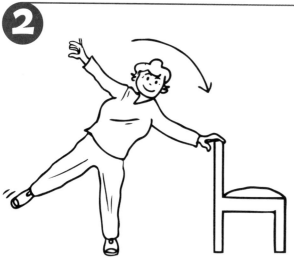

2

2. Lean a little bit to the left while straightening your right leg out to the side for balance. Remember not to lift your right leg too high.

3. Bend your knee again as you return to your starting position.

4. Now repeat the routine with your left leg while leaning to the right.

REPETITIONS: 2 times.

Balance Exercise #23

Lean Into It

This is a very advanced balance exercise.

FOR STARTERS: Hang loose. Big smile. Don't forget to breathe normally.

1. Stand tall, hands resting on your shoulders.

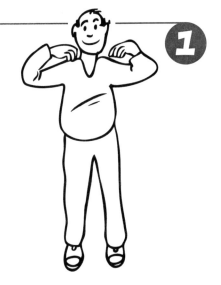

2. Simultaneously, bring left knee up and move arms out to shoulder level.

(continued on next page)

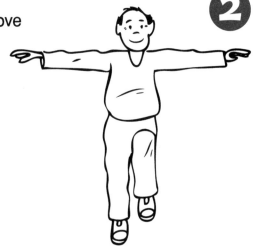

Lean Into It

(continued from previous page)

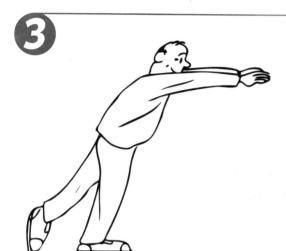

3. Slowly lean forward as your left leg stretches out behind you and both hands reach out in front of you.

4. The first time you do the exercise (or until you feel comfortable) rest your left foot on the floor behind you.

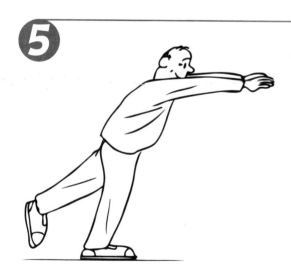

5. When you feel comfortable with the exercise, lift your foot just a few inches off the floor.

Balance Exercise #24

Spin Cycle

This exercise requires your "thinking cap."

FOR STARTERS: Stand tall, feet slightly apart and arms at sides.

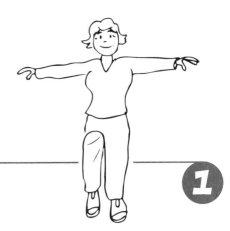

1. Raise your right knee so your foot is just off the floor. Lift your arms out to the side at shoulder level.

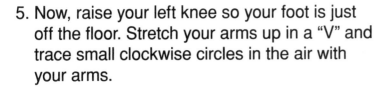

2. Trace small clockwise circles in the air.

3. Lower your right leg and arms, then relax.

4. Using your left leg, repeat steps 1, 2 and 3.

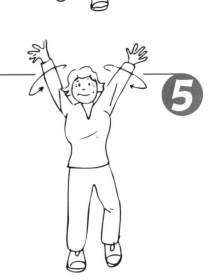

5. Now, raise your left knee so your foot is just off the floor. Stretch your arms up in a "V" and trace small clockwise circles in the air with your arms.

6. Lower your leg and arms, then relax.

7. Raising your right knee, repeat steps 5 and 6.

REPETITION: 1 time. *(continued on next page)*

Balance Exercise #24

Spin Cycle

(continued from previous page)

ADVANCED VERSION

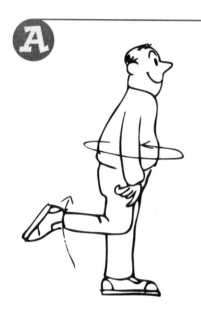

A

1. Bend your left leg at the knee so that your foot is behind you and off the floor. Start with your arms hanging loosely at your sides. Then, gently trace small circles with both arms and left foot.

2. Lower leg and relax.

3. Using your right leg and both arms, repeat steps 1 and 2.

REPETITION: 1 time, or as many as you enjoy!

If you really feel that you're ready for the "Balance Olympics," try the following exercises:

1. With your arms, try tracing circles in the air with both hands going clockwise. Then, try tracing circles with both hands going counterclockwise.

2. Once you've mastered the arms, try tracing clockwise and counterclockwise circles with your raised foot, keeping your arms at your "balance point."

CHAPTER 3
Ball Handling Activities
Balance System Step 3

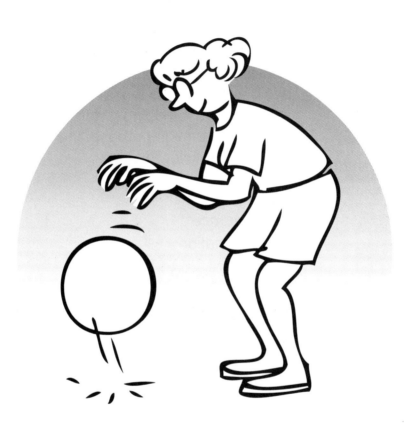

What Is Ball Handling and Why Is It Important?

Ball Handling Activities are fun and easy to do

Ball Handling Activities of the Six-Step Balance System™ are designed to reposition the body constantly in a non-threatening way to develop movement patterns and help stabilize the body.

Over the years, we have proven that Ball Handling Activities are great in many ways: they'll help you avoid negative thinking, and the best news is, you will have fun doing them! The Ball Handling Activities are multi-purpose and help individuals develop the following skills:

Simple Ball Handling Activities provide many benefits

- Body Balance
- Endurance
- Coordination
- Agility
- Lateral Balance
- Leg Strength
- Locomotor Skills
- Relaxation
- Self-Awareness
- Spatial Awareness
- Spatial Relationship
- Visual Response
- Kinesthetic Awareness
- Eye/Hand Coordination
- Gross Motor Coordination
- Visual Motor Coordination
- Figure-Ground Relationship

A leading expert in corrective and high-performance exercise, Paul Chek, founder of the CHEK Institute, says, "Constantly repositioning the body keeps it naturally aware of its surroundings. The movements aren't necessarily planned, and success is based on stabilization, control and trials, not necessarily reps and sets." [14]

Chek goes on to say, "Some of the most effective training for body awareness takes place in more frequent, quicker exposures to challenging activities rather than long durations of practice."

Ball Handling Activities are quick, fun and simple. Each activity requires concentration and accurate response. Ball Handling Activities are great for balance and a fun way to take your mind off problems! In fact, the activities function as a form of non-conventional therapy that will help you balance without thinking.

Ball Handling Activities can help you to become more aware of how you position your body (forward, backward, sideways) and how fast you can move your body.

In addition, by routinely using Ball Handling Activities, you should become more aware of what it feels like to move your arms and feet when you feel you are about to fall; this awareness will also train you to regain balance even more quickly!

Constant repositioning of the body keeps it naturally aware of its surroundings

Balance without thinking

Practice to regain your balance

Once you have practiced Ball Handling Activities for a while, and begin to FEEL what it is like to lean forward, backward or sideways without falling, you will have learned how to reduce your chances of falling and how to reduce injuries in the event of a fall.

We forget the importance of PLAY! The physical experience of bouncing balls is "hands-on," which is fun and at the same time, gives us a "tool" to utilize in fall prevention.

In a speech, Dr. Walter F. Drew, co-founder of the Reusable Resource Association and the Institute for Self Active Education, said, "By playing as adults, by ourselves, or in collaboration with others, we learn again to value the play and creative energy of children." [15]

DR. BETTY'S FITNOTE™

"We don't stop playing because we grow old; we grow old because we stop playing."

– George Bernard Shaw, Literary critic, playwright and essayist. 1925 Nobel Prize for Literature (1856-1950)

Ball Handling Activity #1
Easy Toss Up & Over

You may prefer a larger ball than what is shown.

1. With a ball in either your right or left hand, keep your hands close together.

2. Begin by gently **passing** the ball back and forth from one hand to the other.

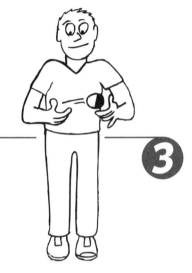

3. Now, **toss** the ball from one hand to the other. Start with your hands very close together; then as you become more confident, move your hands farther and farther apart.

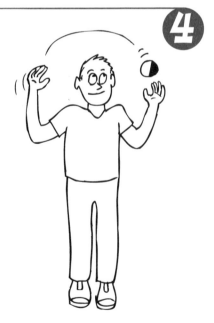

4. Starting again with your hands close together, toss ball up in the air, then catch it. As you become more and more capable, continue to throw the ball higher and higher, as you move your hands farther and farther apart.

As you repeat the exercise, try to sway your body a little from side to side as you toss and catch. Be aware of the shifting of your weight.

Ball Handling Activity #2
Dropsy

Fun to do with music.

1. Hold a ball in your right hand at eye level.

2. Place your left hand underneath your right hand at waist level.

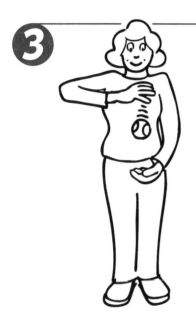

3. Drop the ball into your left hand.

4. Now switch; place your left hand (with the ball) at eye level and your right hand underneath at waist level.

5. Drop the ball into your right hand.

6. Alternate between hands.

7. Slowly increase the distance between your right hand and left hand.

DR. BETTY'S
FITNOTE™

"It is the greatest of all mistakes to do nothing because you can only do a little. Do what you can." – Sydney Smith, English essayist (1771-1845)

Ball Handling Activity #3
Righty/Lefty

Marching music is great for this exercise.

FOR STARTERS: Make sure that the ball has sufficient bounce.

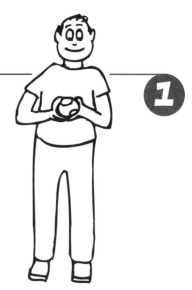

1. Hold the ball with both hands, then say to your-self: "Drop, then catch, then hold."

2. Bounce the ball and eliminate holding it; keep catching and bouncing it 6 to 10 times with both hands.

3. Then bounce the ball with just your right hand 8 to 10 times, then bounce with just your left hand 8 to 10 times.

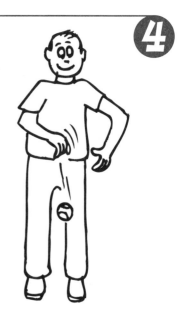

4. Then bounce it with your right hand; as the ball comes back up, catch it and bounce it with your left hand.

Continue bouncing the ball, alternating between right hand and left hand.

DR. BETTY'S FITNOTE™

> **"You grow up the day you have the first real laugh at yourself."**
>
> **– Ethel Barrymore, American Actress (1879-1959)**

Ball Handling Activity #4

3 Levels

Grandchildren love this one.

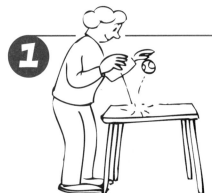

1. Drop and catch the ball on the tabletop 5 times.

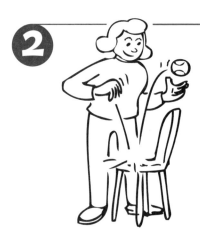

2. Drop and catch the ball on the seat of the kitchen chair 5 times.

3. Next, drop and catch the ball on the kitchen floor 5 times.

4. Now, perform it in a series: drop and catch on the table 1 time, then drop and catch on the seat of the chair 1 time, and drop and catch on the floor 1 time.

Repeat as often as you wish.

Ball Handling Activity #5
Target Practice

Enjoy by having a family contest with this one.

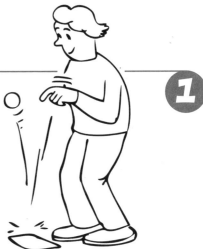

1. Pick a target (e.g. a line or a square on the linoleum or hardwood floor) or make a target out of paper, such as a square, triangle or oval, taped to the floor.

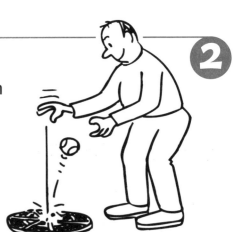

2. Drop the ball on the center of your target. Try and drop the ball "dead center," just as in darts. (If you have a dart target at home, try placing it on the floor and bouncing the ball, hitting the numbers and keeping score.)

DR. BETTY'S
FITNOTE™

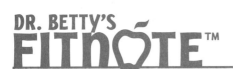

> "We must believe in ourselves or no one else will believe in us; we must match our aspirations with the competence, courage, and determination to succeed."
>
> – Rosalyn Sussman Yalow, Medical physicist, the second woman to win the Nobel Prize in Medicine (1921-)

Ball Handling Activity #6
Travel'n Man

This exercise is easier when you count out loud.

1. Bounce and catch the ball 1 time, then stop.

2. Take one step forward (step with right foot and then bring left foot even with right), then bounce and catch the ball 2 times, then stop.

3. Take two steps forward, then bounce and catch the ball 3 times, then stop.

4. See how many times you can bounce and catch the ball before you find yourself chasing the ball (this is also a great form of exercise).

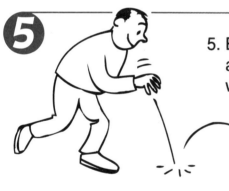

5. Bounce and catch the ball from one room to another, or outside from one end of the driveway to the other.

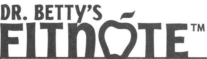

DR. BETTY'S
FITNOTE™

> **"Just don't give up trying to do what you really want to do. Where there is love and inspiration, I don't think you can go wrong."**
>
> **– Ella Fitzgerald, American Jazz singer (1918-1996)**

Ball Handling Activity #7

Playing Catch

Fun to intermingle with children and adults.

1. Stand face to face with your partner and toss the ball back and forth.

2. As you get more comfortable, move farther and farther apart.

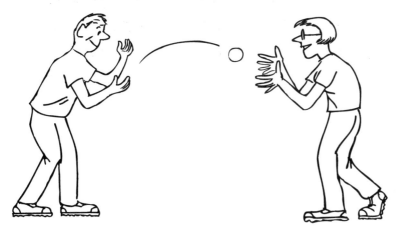

3. You can have a lot of fun with your grandchildren by having them stand between you. Throw the ball to the child, and have the child throw it to your partner. Then, keep it going back and forth.

4. Tape a target on the floor between you and your partner. Bounce the ball off the target so it bounces up toward your partner. For a real challenge, move farther and farther away from the target.

Ball Handling Activity #8
Variations

Try any or all of the variations below.

When you feel comfortable, try adding any of the challenges below to any of the preceding Ball Handling Activities.

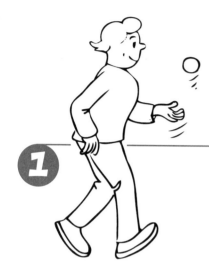

1. Bounce and catch the ball with only your fingertips (instead of the palm of your hand).

2. Toss the ball, clap once. Toss the ball, clap twice.

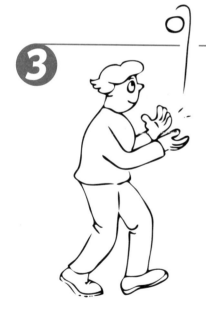

3. Bounce and catch the ball with both hands as you walk on your "balance beam."

4. Bounce and catch the ball while you *look* at a "target" that is at eye level. Then *walk* toward that target while continuing to bounce the ball.

5. Start slowly, then increase walking and bouncing speed; then decrease speed.

6. Bounce ball while walking sideways, varying your starting position by alternating your right and left feet.

CHAPTER 4
Walking While Talking
on the Phone
Balance System Step 4

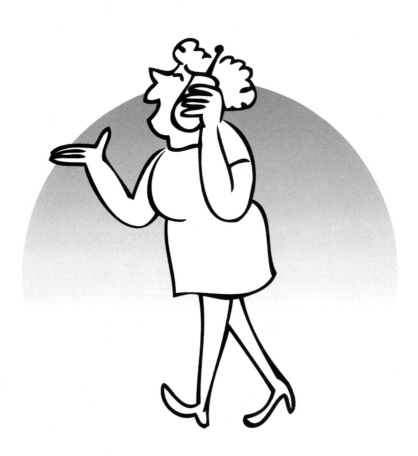

What Is Walking While Talking on the Phone and Why Is It Important?

Walking is one of the best types of exercise

One of the most efficient and familiar activities that promote overall fitness of the body is walking. That's right, walking!

Therefore, it is important to understand how walking and balance work together. Without question, the act of walking requires good balance, and good balance requires that one must walk!

To help achieve this goal, I have included walking as part of the Six-Step Balance System,™ using an approach known as Walking While Talking on the Phone. Walk as far as your phone line allows.

The primary objective of this exercise activity is to help you practice what is known as "dual-tasking." Simply put, you will be performing two events at the same time: namely, "walking" while "talking" on the phone.

Think about it: The ability to walk without thinking is a unique human skill

An individual's position in space depends totally on the ability to overcome gravity and remain balanced. As a result, it is important for everyone to continue developing the skill of balancing their bodies. The ability to walk securely, without thinking about walking, is a unique human skill.

A good deal of movement relies on having healthy feet and good leg muscles. The more fit the feet and legs are, the more a body can resist falls. The feet and legs provide a steady foundation on which balancing activities are based.

While walking and talking can make anyone "huff and puff" if they are not in shape, walking and talking remains a great way to improve balance.

Whether long or short conversations, phone calls can now become a partner in your daily exercise routine. Walking not only contributes to improving the cardiovascular system, it also acts as an overall body toner and strengthener.

Strong legs make it easier to get up from a chair

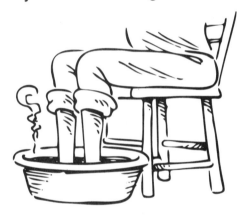

DR. BETTY'S FITNŌTE™

"The sovereign invigorator of the body is exercise, and of all the exercises walking is the best."

– Thomas Jefferson, 3rd U.S. President (1801-09), one of the authors of the Declaration of Independence (1762-1826)

*Don't forget
the importance
of having good
posture*

Perhaps one of the most overlooked aspects of daily health and fitness is posture. In addition to its medical benefits, good posture says a lot about who we are and how we feel. We all remember being told at a young age by a teacher or parent to "Stand up straight. Throw your shoulders back and stop slouching."

Well, the advice is as good now as it was then. So, when you are "Walking and Talking" on the phone, stand up as straight as possible and keep that smile in your voice!

*It's never too
late to improve
one's posture*

Good news — it's never too late to improve one's posture. Dr. Pauline Camacho, director of Loyola University's Osteoporosis and Metabolic Bone Disease Center, says "Even patients with mild osteoporosis can make dramatic improvements with a series of posture exercises." [16]

Posture exercises can be fun. For starters, try the two exercises below:

Wall Arch

1. Face a wall at arms length and feet 6 inches apart.

2. Stretch your arms out in front, at shoulder height, touch the wall, then take a deep breath and hold.

3. Flatten your stomach; exhale as you lower your arms to your sides.

Start with 3 repetitions per day. Gradually work your way up to whatever feels good to you.

Midback Posture Correction

1. Sit on a chair with your chin tucked inward.

2. Keep your stomach tight, chest forward and feet together (flat on the floor).

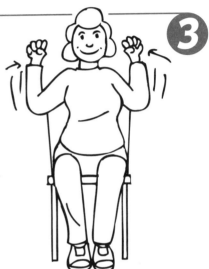

3. Place your arms in a "W" position with your shoulders relaxed (not hunched) and elbows bent.

4. Bring the elbows back, gently squeezing the shoulder blades together.

5. Hold for a slow count of 3; then relax for a slow count of 3.

Start with 3 repetitions per day. Work up to 5 repetitions per day.

DR. BETTY'S FITNOTE™

"There is so much to gain from improving your posture. Everybody's interested in the way they look, and then they're astounded to find the other benefits."

- Janice Novak, author, speaker and wellness consultant

Poor posture can aggravate arthritic conditions and/or cause muscle spasms and chronic back pain. They may all lead to improper breathing.

Practice good posture when you are walking and sitting. Remember that good posture is the basis of good health. Always begin walking exercises or activities with this in mind.

Practice good posture when you're standing or sitting

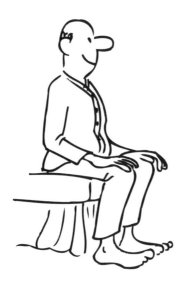

DR. BETTY'S FITNOTE™

"I grew up to have my father's looks, my father's speech patterns, my father's posture, my father's opinions and my mother's contempt for my father."

– Jules Feiffer, American cartoonist, novelist, playwright, and screen writer (1929-)

Recommendation #3

Dressing for Comfort

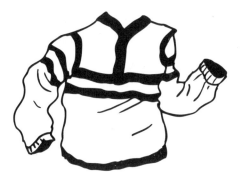

Dress comfortably, especially if you are walking outdoors. Your exercise clothing should be loose-fitting to allow for freedom of movement. As a rule of thumb, wear lighter clothes than temperatures warrant. Exercise generates a great deal of body heat, so be sure to dress in "layers," so as you build up body heat you can take off a sweater or jacket, along the way.

On cold days, always wear a hat to prevent loss of body heat. On hot, sunny days, wearing a hat that provides some shade is also a good idea. In warm climates or seasons, walking or other outdoor exercises should be done during the coolest parts of the day, early morning or after sunset.

Also, never wear rubberized or plastic clothing. Such garments interfere with the evaporation of perspiration and can cause body temperature to rise to dangerous levels fairly quickly. Always, regardless of the weather, remember to drink lots of water to avoid dehydration.

Another tip is to turn your socks inside out so the seams (if there are any) do not rub against your feet and cause discomfort. Remember to keep your toe nails trimmed. They can also be a "sore spot" for walkers! Again, we want to remind you of the importance of wearing comfortable, flat shoes when walking. Sneakers with good arch supports are your best bet.

Walking Warm-Up Exercise #1
Just Leaning Around

Before walking anywhere, warm-up by stretching.

FOR STARTERS: WARM UP FIRST! You'll avoid shin-splints and strained heel cords. Also, whenever possible don't drive the car, don't take the bus, don't get a ride...walk!

1. With your back straight and your feet together, stand an arm's length away from a wall; keep your heels on the floor.

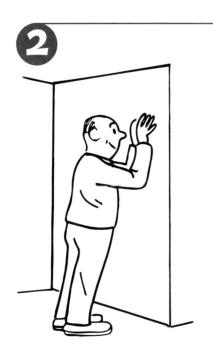

2. Bend your elbows so your forearms "lean" against the wall.

3. Hold the bent arm position for 5 to 10 seconds. (Remember to keep your heels flat on the floor!) Feel your leg muscles stretch.

4. Relax and repeat as often as you feel necessary. (Some people find they like doing this exercise in the morning, again at noon, and then just before going to bed at night.)

Get off the bus before your stop and walk! Walk to the store! Wear out the rugs at home! Use the stairs! (Start with one flight; then gradually increase the number of flights.) Substitute a quick walk down the block for one of your favorite (too rich) desserts!

Walking Warm-Up Exercise #2
Jamb Session

To avoid leg cramps, drink lots of water.

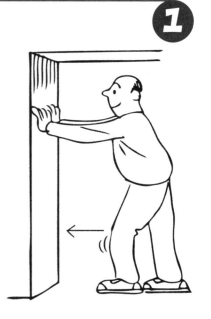

1. Holding onto a door jamb, place your right foot directly behind the left (with toes of right foot touching heel of left foot and right heel flat on the floor).

2. Now, bend your left knee slightly and feel the stretch in your right leg. Hold for a count of 5.

3. Straighten and return to starting position.

4. Relax, then repeat with other leg, placing your left foot directly behind your right foot. Hold for another count of 5.

Change foot positions a minimum of 2 times. If you suffer from periodic leg cramps, perform this exercise as often as needed.

DR. BETTY'S FITNOTE™

As you age, you become more susceptible to dehydration for several reasons: Your body's ability to conserve water is reduced, your thirst sense becomes less acute and you're less able to respond to changes in temperature.[17] — MayoClinic.com

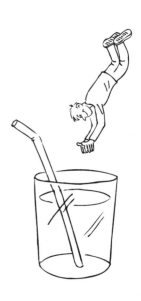

Everyday walking has many benefits

Walking is an activity that doesn't really have to be learned. And our normal, everyday walking pattern is the perfect way to get started on the road to fitness and better balance. There are so many opportunities to "build the benefits" of walking — from gradually increasing the frequency to increasing the pace.

After you've started walking, try adding some fun (and flexibility for your legs, ankles, feet, and toes) with a few of the walking variations my friends and I are doing. I'll admit, people sometimes wonder what we're up to, but I'll bet their balance and muscle tone don't hold a candle to ours!

Remember to rest occasionally

As you're walking, pay attention to keeping your chin in, chest up and shoulders back (with your hips in line under your shoulders). Your knees should be relaxed and your abdomen should be pulled in (toward an imaginary wall behind you).

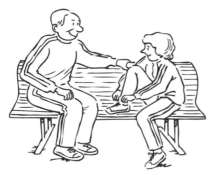

DR. BETTY'S FITNOTE™

"One step at a time is good walking."

– Confucius, China's most famous teacher, philosopher and political theorist (551-479 BC)

Walking Warm-Up Exercise #3
Side-Step The Issue

This exercise increases hip flexibility.

Here's one occasion when sidestepping is a dandy way to get ahead. Just be careful how far you go.

Next time you're out (or in!) walking, stop and then go to the right with a sideways step (or slide).

1. Start with your right, then bring your left foot to meet (and touch) it.

2. Step - close - step - close, until you've reached the curb or wall or any other "barrier."

3. Now, sidestep to the left, back onto your original path and continue your regular walk.

Play it cool. People will definitely wonder whether you're a clever pantomimist or just stuck on some bubble gum!

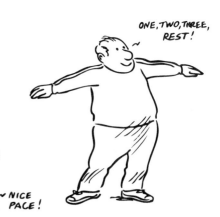

Walking Warm-Up Exercise #4
Zig and Zag

Did you know that pretending reduces stress?

Use your imagination! Every time you walk, spend a few minutes pretending you're negotiating some difficult "terrain." You'll vary your pace and have a good laugh, too, probably at some spectator's expense!

1

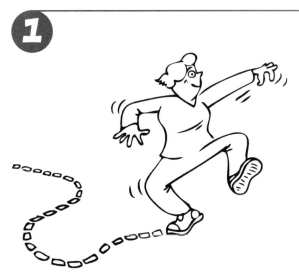

1. Walk in a zig-zag pattern.

2. Now, wiggle your body while you walk.

3. Now, walk like a robot.

4. Walk "heavy," then walk "light."

   Here's a fun variation of "Zig and Zag" that will strengthen your ankles and test your balance:

5. Walk 4 steps forward on the balls of your feet, keeping your heels slightly elevated.

Walking Warm-Up Exercise #5
Spring Fling

This exercise is a great aide for improving posture.

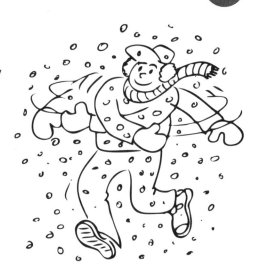

1. As you walk, "fling" your arms across your chest, then out to the side in rhythmic repetitions.

2. 8 flings (across and out) should do it every time you walk.

I said "spring" because it rhymes! You can do this any season of the year.

Walking Warm-Up Exercise #6
Skater's Waltz

Your shoulders will say "thank you."

1. Bring your arms comfortably behind your lower back, then clasp your hands together and stretch your arms as much as you can.

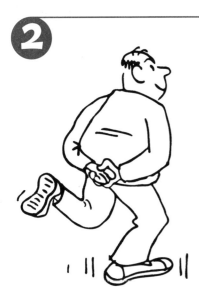

2. Pull your arms down and walk as if you were skating for 10 to 20 steps. (As soon as you try this, you'll remember your smoothest glides across the ice.)

3. Relax your arms; shake them loose. Then, repeat 2 or 3 times.

DR. BETTY'S FITNOTE™

> "If you haven't exercised for a long time, just start out for a couple of minutes a day. Then work it up a little bit. You'd be surprised at the end of thirty days, how many things you are doing."
> — Jack LaLanne, fitness guru (1914-)

Walking is a great way to meet new people and enjoy the company of others who are as interested as you are in fitness, better balance and fun. One super place to find your contemporaries and have your daily walk is in a shopping mall. (And for once, you don't have to buy a thing!) In fact, lots of seniors now go to malls just to get in shape.

What could be better, after all? Malls are climate controlled, safe and spacious. Some malls open early for walkers. Others have clubs to bring walkers together. Stop by one of your local malls and ask about their provisions for walking.

Wherever you plan your walk for health, don't waste another minute. Start now!

Happy Walking! Keep Smiling!

Walking is a great way to meet new people

Whether it's Walking While Talking on the Phone, or in the mall, get walking today!

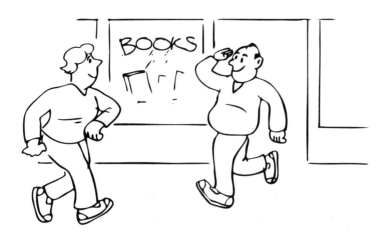

CHAPTER 5
The '10 Martini' Slump
Balance System Step 5

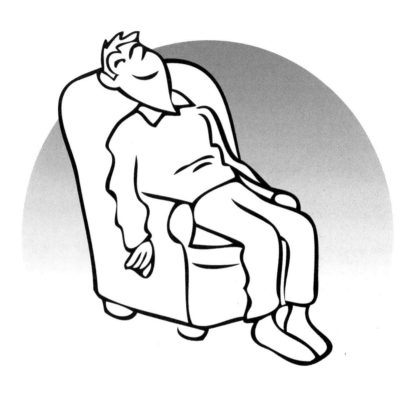

What Is "The Slump" and Why Is It Important?

How to practice falling the safe way

Have you ever practiced falling? Probably not.

As a result, if you had fallen, you no doubt tensed your body, became very rigid and suffered an injury. Of course, we all know that serious injuries to older adults could mean the end of their mobility and independence.

The Slump used to be known as "The Ten Martini Slump." (I used this name because of its vivid imagery, but decided to change it because it implied heavy consumption of alcohol, which I do not advocate.)

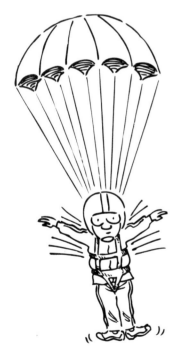

As an integral part of the Six-Step Balance System,™ The Slump enables a person to slump and experience total body relaxation while learning "how to fall."

Loss of balance is a serious problem for many seniors. The Slump exercises simulate a person with a loss of balance, but under conscious and thoughtful conditions.

People who have practiced slumping don't resist when they fall. What they are doing, in fact, is training what is clinically known as their proprioceptive sense, which is one's ability to sense their bone joint position and joint motion.

This proprioceptive sense, which I like to call the "sixth sense" is trainable. Use of the Six-Step Balance System™ has proven that a well-trained sixth sense helps to prevent falls and reduce serious injuries from falls.

Learn to train your "sixth sense"

One of my favorite syndicated columnists, Dr. Paul Donohue, in a popular article on balance once wrote: "If you could only react quickly enough to straighten the ankle, you might avoid the sprain. Unfortunately, it is difficult to react quickly enough by 'thinking,' midway in a fall, to stop falling!" [18]

So then, what can make the difference? What can help you react quickly enough to prevent falls and injuries? One answer that has been discovered is to train your sixth sense continually by practicing the "Art of Falling." This will enable you to react at the subconscious level.

You can practice the "art of falling" to reduce injury

In other words, you will be functioning on what I call "automatic pilot." You will react quickly and correctly without the complex and time consuming thought process Dr. Donohue spoke of.

We have observed that in the event of a fall, the well-trained proprioceptive sense allows you to instinctively relax and slump into the fall, avoiding serious injury.

Use your chair and bed to practice The Slump

As Dr. Donohue further stated, "The proprioceptive sense is what controls the correct position of the body in relationship to its surroundings. In the human body, the proprioceptive sense is like the sensing equipment in a spaceship that controls altitude, direction, etc., during liftoff and landing."

For certain, no matter how careful you are, there may be times when an accidental fall may occur. So, be prepared for it! The Slump instructs you how to use your chair and bed to fall safely.

The more you practice falling, the more functional the sixth sense becomes. As a result, your body will be trained to remain loose and flexible.

A stiff body breaks! A limp body bends!

Remember, a stiff body breaks, a limp body bends. You can avoid broken bones! **Please practice every day!**

DR. BETTY'S FITNOTE™

The body must function at a subconscious level. There is no time during a fall to say to yourself, "I have to do this, this and this." You MUST be on automatic pilot.

How To Fall Safely Exercise #1
The Slump: Into the Chair

This exercise can be a lifesaver!

FOR STARTERS: You will be very successful with The Slump, if you always remember to "hang loose." Wiggle your buttocks, shake out your arms and legs, take a deep breath and exhale with a long, relaxing sigh.

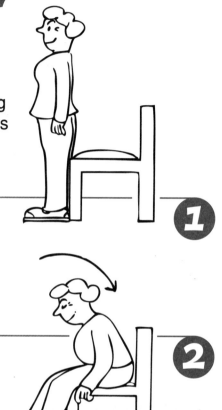

1. Stand tall in front of a stationary chair, with the seat brushing the backs of your legs. Feet should be a comfortable distance apart and arms should be hanging loosely at your sides.

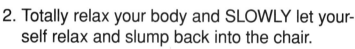

2. Totally relax your body and SLOWLY let yourself relax and slump back into the chair.

3. Slump your shoulders and do your best "rag doll" impression!

REPETITIONS: Every time you sit down to read or watch TV, have a contest with your friends. Who has the most relaxed Slump?

REMEMBER: You will not have time to think "relax and let go." You must have trained your mind and body to fall loose.

How To Fall Safely Exercise #2
The Slump: Into the Bed

This exercise must be performed daily!

FOR STARTERS: Special Alert!!! Please, **DO NOT** go to bed without performing The Slump!

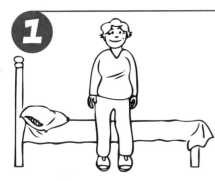

1. You should be standing in the center of the side of your bed, with your back toward the bed. Stand tall, feet comfortably apart with the backs of your legs touching the bed and arms hanging loosely at your sides.

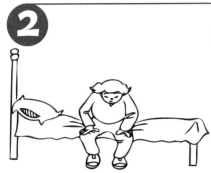

2. Bending at the knees, SLOWLY and very loosely collapse into a sitting position on the bed. Slump your shoulders and relax your entire body during this simulated "fall."

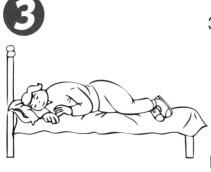

3. Now, collapse on either your left shoulder and side or right shoulder and side (whichever bed-side you started on with your head toward the headboard). Still remaining as loose and limber as possible, bring your knees up slightly toward your chest.

REPETITIONS: Every time you go to bed or lie down for a nap.

CHAPTER 6
Dancing with a Pillow
Balance System Step 6

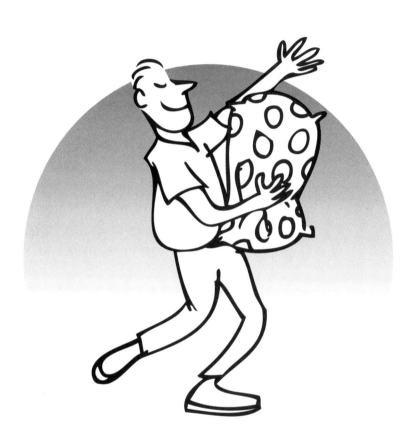

What Is Dancing With A Pillow And Why Is It Important?

Dancing is a fun and viable form of exercise

Is dancing a viable form of exercise? You bet it is!

To access this easy form of exercise, I included Dancing with a Pillow as a major component of the Six-Step Balance System.™ This effective training and conditioning technique will help seniors prevent falls.

It would be wonderful if we could wave a magic wand over our loved ones to prevent falls. We cannot. But, we can give them a resource, not only to prevent falls but also to strengthen legs and heart and improve balance, coordination and posture. At the same time, they will have fun!

That resource is their pillow, and the method is Dancing with a Pillow to their favorite waltz or any other dance style.

Dancing allows you to move in many directions

When I ask seniors to walk backward, rigor mortis sets in. Yet, when Dancing with a Pillow, they are moving not only forward and backward but also sideways and in circles. Foot patterns are simple at first, but become very complex as the music goes on. Remember, they have removed one arm, a *stabilizer*. As they continue dancing, I ask them to change hands, right arm on pillow, left hand up. A few minutes later, I ask them to hold the pillow against their chest with both hands.

Now we have removed *both* stabilizers. Dancing with a Pillow, they are on their own with no partner for bodily support.

SIDENOTE:

In the summer of 2004, at a senior outing, I asked 121 seniors to dance with their paper plates, acting as their pillow. At the end of the *Tennessee Waltz,* a gentleman who was 82 years young came up to me and said, "Betty, don't tell my wife, but I was dancing with my first love."

Let's dance in another time, another place

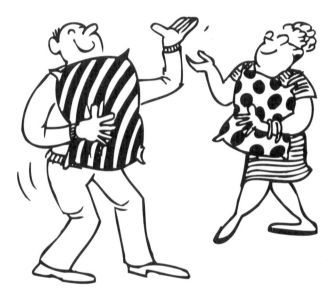

Remember, the desire to reminisce is important in today's virtual world.

Not everyone can go outside during the winter, but anyone can dance with a pillow every day. And when you're having a family dinner, after you finished, invite them into another room, put on your favorite music and enjoy an inter-generational "pillow dance."

Dancing with a Pillow creates an environment that reduces fear. It is significant in achieving muscle relaxation and the activation of a healthy and motivating state of memory recall.

Without question, practicing the combination of Dancing with a Pillow and the exercises from the Six-Step Balance System™ can have a positive and significant impact on reducing falls and the debilitating injuries they cause.

Many additional benefits of dancing – increased flexibility, coordination and overall well being – have also been documented. Dancers develop strong muscles, improved coordination, agility and balance.

Dancing can be used as a weight maintenance program if practiced faithfully. Dancing strengthens muscles not used in other activities because it requires movement in different directions and with varying speeds.

DR. BETTY'S
FITNOTE™

Dancing can be magical and transforming. It can breathe new life into a tired soul... dancing can give you a great mind-body workout. [19] – AARP

Because it is low impact, dancing is generally easier to tolerate for some people who have orthopedic concerns.

Dancing has been shown to increase bone density and help prevent osteoporosis, which is a process not an event. Some 25 million Americans, 80% of them women, have osteoporosis.[20] It is also affecting men in increasing numbers.

A favorite song can stay with you for days and bring a smile long after the last note. Dancing is a great opportunity to get away from the pressures of daily work or other obligations. It can make you walk taller.

In addition, dancing fits easily within one's schedule. As neuro-ophthalmologist Dr. David N. Smith noted, "The problem is when you are busy, it's hard to find time to exercise, and that's what's nice about dancing. It's physical and it's pleasurable."[21]

Dancing to familiar tunes takes us back to very pleasant times and places

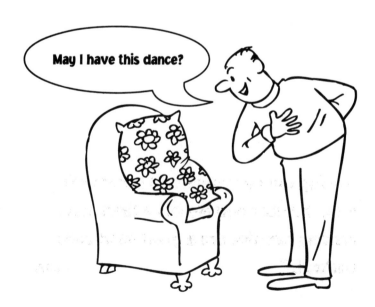

Social dancing can help you burn up to 250 calories an hour

According to the American Council of Exercise, social dancers can burn up to 250 calories per hour.[22] In addition to the physical benefits, some dancers have said dancing just makes them feel young again! I also strongly believe that music plays a large part in these emotions.

In fact, Plato once said, "Music gives a soul to the universe, wings to the mind, flight to the imagination, a charm to sadness, gaiety and life to everything."

Music is like medicine

As an added benefit of Dancing with a Pillow, exciting new research suggests that the human brain responds to music almost as if it were medicine. In addition, through my years of experience and careful observations, I have found an increased energy level in participants after they have danced.

Slower dances like the fox-trot or waltz aren't necessarily aerobic, but they can help you develop strength and improve balance and posture.

"Everyone needs to exercise. If you do something you like doing, you're likely to stick with it," says Joseph Phillips, a senior and former Marine Corps veteran from Washington D.C., who dances to help control his hypertension.

As mentioned previously, the Six-Step Balance System™ gives individuals a proven resource not only to prevent falls, but also to strengthen legs and heart; to improve balance, coordination and posture; and, at the same time, have fun!

I would like to close this chapter with a poem by Mark Twain that I think you will like:

> *Dance like nobody's watching;*
>
> *Love like you can't be hurt.*
>
> *Sing like nobody's listening;*
>
> *Live like it's heaven on earth.*[23]

Dancing is also a great way to relieve stress

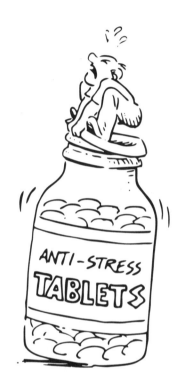

DR. BETTY'S FITNOTE™

Dancing provides many benefits. Wherever you are in your physical ability, just swaying to some of your favorite songs while remaining balanced will help your body and mind.

Afterword

I think we have covered a number of important issues in this book. We have known for some time that falling, and the thoughts of the real dangers of falling, have forced fear and inactivity into the lives of many of our ever-growing senior population.

We have the power to make better choices about our health

Fortunately, this very real problem no longer needs to be true. Within recent years, we have begun to discover that we can help prevent a lot of problems in our lives by making better choices when it comes to our health. For instance, by conquering our fears and practicing the Six-Step Balance System,™ we can actually minimize and in many cases reduce the risks of falling.

As I described earlier, I have seen remarkable changes in every one of my students. And what has been true for them can be true for you! All it takes is your determination and your commitment to setting and achieving your goals. Remember, the benefits to be gained from making the Six-Step Balance System™ part of your daily routine go far beyond preventing any falls.

Given the unpredictable nature of falls and how falls can interrupt the natural balance system, keep in mind that, if properly trained, the brain and the body can interact to fall more safely.

Without question, such information becomes very important when developing techniques on how to anticipate falls and how to fall more safely; and more importantly, how to train the human body to balance better and skillfully in order to prevent falls.

Movement and exercise decrease the problems associated with such physical disorders as arthritis, osteoporosis, high blood pressure and heart disease. In addition, they also improve your mental, emotional and social well-being.

You can't go wrong taking care of yourself using the Six-Step Balance System.™ Age is not a factor! You can exercise some control over the quality of your life. So start today!

Make preventing falls a part of your daily life

DR. BETTY'S FITNOTE™

"Age is an issue of mind over matter.

If you don't mind, it doesn't matter."

– Mark Twain, American humorist, writer and lecturer (1835-1910)

APPENDIX

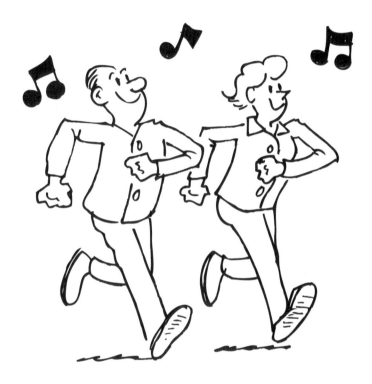

"May you always walk in the sunshine of life."
–Betty Perkins-Carpenter, Ph.D.

Contract with Myself

Recognizing the benefits of The Six-Step Balance System,™ especially how this important series of exercise activities can help me prevent falls, I agree to the following as part of a new contract with myself:

- I'll set my sights on doing everything within my power to reduce my fear of falling, prevent falls and, if a fall is inevitable, learn how to fall to limit possible injury.

- I'll talk about The Six-Step Balance System™ with my doctor so she/he can further advise me.

- I'll be realistic in the goals that I set for myself.

- I'll keep track of my progress along the way.

- I'll remain faithful to The Six-Step Balance System™ and promise not to give up on myself.

- I'll encourage everyone I know to discover The Six-Step Balance System.™

- I'll share this contract with my family and friends in order to gain their support and encouragement.

- I'll remember that one of the most important contracts I have in life is this contract with myself!

Signature _____ Date _____

Fall-Proofing Your Home: Checklist
Lighting

	Yes	No

Can you turn on a light without having to walk into a dark room? You should always turn on lights before going into a room, even if you are going in for a moment.

Do you move slowly when lighting is dim, giving your eyes time to adjust between well-lit and dark areas?

Do you replace burnt-out bulbs immediately?

Do you have night lights in your hallways, bedrooms, stairwells and living areas? Nightlights are inexpensive and invaluable for visibility at night, particularly in stairwells, hallways, bathrooms and bedrooms.

Do you keep a flashlight by your bed? Be sure to check the battery frequently.

Are there lights and light switches installed at both the top and bottom of the stairways?

Is the lighting bright but not creating glare?

Do you wear sunglasses during bright days or around ice and snow to reduce blinding glare?

Fall-Proofing Your Home: Checklist
Walkways

yes   no

☐ ☐ **Do you use non-skid wax, or no wax at all, on polished floors?**

☐ ☐ **Are walkways kept clear of things that could trip you, such as cords, low furniture and toys?** Tape cords to the floor or wall. Tie up extra cord with a rubber band, or coil it up inside an empty toilet paper tube.

☐ ☐ **Do you immediately replace breaks in linoleum, broken floorboards, or flooring that is buckling?**

☐ ☐ **Do you clean up spills on floors immediately?**

☐ ☐ **Do you arrange your furniture in each room so that a clear and wide walking lane is left open?** Make wide turns when you are walking around corners.

☐ ☐ **Does your favorite chair have arm rests that are long enough to help you get up and sit down?**

☐ ☐ **Are your chairs and tables stable enough to support your weight if you lean on them?**

☐ ☐ **Are your outdoor stairs and walkways free from cracks, dips and holes?**

Fall-Proofing Your Home: Checklist
Stairways

	yes	no
Can you clearly see the outline of each step as you go both up and down? Each step can be marked with brightly colored adhesive tape strips. Don't use shag carpets, deep-piled carpets or carpets with busy patterns on stairs.	☐	☐
Do all stairways have securely-fixed handrails on both sides? Rails should extend beyond the top and bottom steps and the ends should turn in. If you should start to fall, do not let go of the railing: hang on!	☐	☐
Does your hand wrap easily and completely around the rail? Rails should be round and anchored one to two inches away from walls.	☐	☐
Are all carpets and runners well-fastened down? Use double-sided tape or carpet tacks. Repair holes in carpeting. Get rid of frayed rugs.	☐	☐
Do stairs have even surfaces (no metal strips or rubber mats to trip you up)?	☐	☐
Are stairs kept free of clutter?	☐	☐
Can you reach the things you use most often without using a step-stool?	☐	☐

Fall-Proofing Your Home: Checklist
Bathroom

Yes	no	
☐	☐	**Do the tub and shower have rubber mats, non-skid strips or non-skid surfaces?**
☐	☐	**Do you have a grab bar on the wall or side of the tub/shower?** If balance or weakness is a problem, you should use a bath seat.
☐	☐	**Can you get on and off the toilet easily?** If not, you should install a raised toilet seat and fix a grab bar into the wall next to the toilet. Or, install a grab bar that fastens onto the back of the toilet seat.
☐	☐	**Do you always test the tub or shower water to make sure it is not too hot, so that you do not make a quick, reactive movement and lose your balance?**
☐	☐	**If you splash water or suds from the tub onto the floor, do you wipe it up right away?**
☐	☐	**As an added precaution, do you dry yourself off before getting out of the tub or shower?**

Fall-Proofing Your Home: Checklist
General

	yes	no
Do you take time to find your balance when you sit up after lying down, or stand up after sitting?	☐	☐
Do you wear rubber-soled, low-heeled shoes? Do your slippers fit well and have soles that provide traction? Keep the bottom of your shoes clean. Avoid walking in stocking feet or in socks.	☐	☐
If you feel dizzy from time to time, do you use a cane, walking stick, or walker?	☐	☐
Do you watch for slippery pavement when walking outdoors and entering/leaving cars and buses? When walking on slippery or uneven surfaces, lean forward slightly, relax your knees and take shorter steps, or shuffle your steps to keep your center of balance under you.	☐	☐
When carrying packages, do you make sure they don't block your view? Divide large loads into smaller ones, leaving one hand free.	☐	☐
When you get out of a car, do you test the ground for wetness or iciness before standing up and walking? Don't hurry — be wary!	☐	☐
Do you avoid rushing to answer the phone/doorbell?	☐	☐

Fall-Proofing Your Home: Checklist
Other Safety Tips

Always use a step-stool, never a chair, when you have to reach high places.

When coming down extremely narrow steps, feel the back of your leg against the step so you won't slip off. Put your whole foot down and concentrate on each movement as you descend the stairs.

Climb down those steps carefully, especially the last step!

It is extremely important to be aware of the last step! It is very easy to *think* you are on the last step but, if you are not paying attention, you may still be on the second or third step from the bottom. Do not talk to anyone while walking down the steps. And if someone calls to you while descending steps, **DO NOT** turn your head to respond. Wait until you reach the bottom. In your own home, count and memorize the number of steps to be negotiated.

When you visit friends, be alert to possible hazards since you are in an unfamiliar environment. You might consider alerting friends to any problems that they are unaware of in their homes. Be especially careful of entrances with steps and elevations in split-level homes. Use a railing whenever available

Curbs can be dangerous

Curbs can be dangerous. Some are poorly identified, broken, very high and sometimes badly illuminated. Be alert as you enter and exit areas that have curbs. It is so easy to be talking to a friend and not be alert to danger.

Fall-Proofing Your Home: Checklist
Other Safety Tips

(continued from previous page)

Carts in a supermarket can also be a problem. DO NOT WALK BACKWARD even 1, 2, or 3 feet to reach for that can of tuna fish you forgot; it is too easy to lose your balance and fall backward. Take the extra few minutes to go around the aisle.

Do not walk backward

Never, never stand on a chair when you change a light bulb or to reach a high shelf or cabinet. If you must reach a high shelf, purchase a sturdy stepladder.

Have your vision tested regularly. If you have your vision corrected and need new glasses, be very careful until your eyes adjust to the new prescription. Also have your hearing tested regularly. Even the simple task of removing ear wax can improve your balance.

Use caution in getting up too quickly after eating, lying down or resting. Low blood pressure may cause dizziness at these times.

Don't stand up too quickly

Talk to your doctor or pharmacist about the side effects of the drugs you are taking and how they may affect your coordination or balance.

Limit your intake of alcohol. Even a little alcohol can further disturb already impaired balance and reflexes.

Fall-Proofing Your Home: Checklist
Other Safety Tips

(continued from previous page)

Make sure that the nighttime temperature in your home is not lower than 65°F. Prolonged exposure to cold temperatures may cause your body temperature to drop, leading to dizziness and falling. Older people cannot tolerate cold as well as younger people can.

Maintain a regular program of activity

Maintain a regular program of activity. Many people enjoy walking, swimming and exercise. Mild weight-bearing activities may reduce the loss of bone from osteoporosis. It is important, however, to check with your doctor or physical therapist to plan a suitable exercise program.

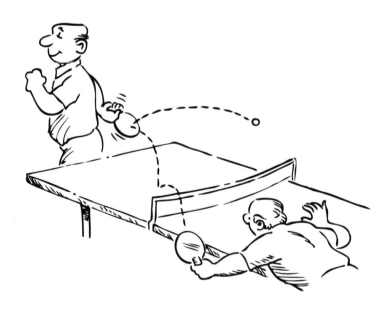

Important Resources & Publications
Website Addresses

A Tool Kit to Prevent Senior Falls: Brochures
Designed for fall prevention programs, *A Tool Kit To Prevent Senior Falls* includes fact sheets, graphs and brochures about falls and fall prevention. (National Center for Injury Prevention and Control)

www.cdc.gov/ncipc/pub-res/toolkit/toolkit.htm

Protecting the Elderly from Falls
Important articles and information on fall statistics and prevention. Articles on how to easily fall-proof your home. (National Safety Council)

www.nsc.org/issues/fallstop.htm

Falls in Older Adults: Management in Primary Practice
Used for the evaluation and management of falls. Includes "Get Up and Go Test," a home safety questionnaire and an evaluation form. Educational materials for patient/family include tips for reducing risk of falls and improving balance. (American Geriatrics Society)

www.americangeriatrics.org/education/falls.shtml

Home Design
Provides help to seniors who wish to stay in their own homes but are facing mobility limitations. This Web page features ideas for making the home more safe and accessible. (AARP)

www.aarp.org/life/homedesign

U.S. Administration on Aging
Search by state to identify state and area agencies on aging.

www.aoa.gov/eldfam/How_To_Find/Agencies/Agencies.asp

(continued from previous page)

Safe Steps Program Materials

The Home Safety Council has developed the national Safe Steps program designed to educate older adults and their family members on how to reduce their risk of falling dangers.

www.homesafetycouncil.org/programs/pr_falls_p000.pdf

The Archstone Foundation

The Archstone foundation is a grant-making organization created to help society meet the needs of the elderly. The site provides publications and useful resources and links to grant projects.

www.archstone.org

The National Council on the Aging

The National Council on the Aging is a national network of organizations and individuals dedicated to improving the health and independence of older persons and increasing their continuing contributions to communities, society and future generations.

www.ncoa.org

WebMD

Offers information, supportive communities and in-depth reference material about health subjects. Board-certified physicians, award-winning journalists, and trained community moderators provide news for the public, up-to-date medical reference content databases, medical imagery, graphics, live web events and interactive tools.

www.webmd.com

Important Resources & Publications
Website Addresses

(continued from previous page)

MedlinePlus
MedlinePlus will direct you to information to help answer health questions. Preformulated MEDLINE searches are included in MedlinePlus and give easy access to medical journal articles. MedlinePlus also has information about drugs, an illustrated medical encyclopedia and the latest health news.

www.medlineplus.gov

FirstGov.Gov
Use this powerful search engine as you look for an ever-growing collection of topical and customer-focused links for seniors. It connects you to millions of web pages – from the federal government, local and tribal governments to foreign nations worldwide.

www.seniors.gov

MayoClinic.com
Provides useful and up-to-date information and tools that reflect the expertise and standard of excellence of Mayo Clinic. A team of Web-publishing professionals and medical experts work side-by-side to produce this site, offering unique access to the experience and knowledge of more than 2,000 physicians and scientists.

www.mayoclinic.com

Thirdage.Com
Provides information relating to relationships, romance, health, wellness, well-being, spirituality and personal growth and development.

www.thirdage.com

Footnotes

1 United States. U.S. Census Bureau, 2004, "U.S. Interim Projections by Age, Sex, Race, and Hispanic Origin," (March 18, 2004), www.census.gov/ipc/www/usinterimproj (January 12, 2006)

2 National Center for Injury Prevention and Control, "A Tool Kit to Prevent Senior Falls," (Sept. 9, 2005), www.cdc.gov/ncipc/pub-res/toolkit/toolkit.htm (November 10, 2005)

3 Yale University School of Medicine, http://ymghealthinfo.org

4 Bob Anderson, www.stretching.com (December 5, 2005)

5 "Falls Free: Promoting A National Falls Prevention Action Plan," (2005), National Council on Aging, www.healthyagingprograms.org (December 13, 2005)

6 Goldberg, Alan, Dr., www.competitivedge.com

7 Whiting, Jim, www.jimtoons.com

8 Williams, Dr. T. Franklin

9 "Stretching Exercises," (2004), National Institute of Health, nihseniorhealth.gov/exercise/stretchingexercises/01.html

10 Thinkexist.com, (2006), www.thinkexist.com

11 MedicineNet.com

12 "Footwear Guide," (2000), American Academy of Orthopedic Surgeons, orthoinfo.aaos.org/fact (July 25, 2005)

13 "Foot and Ankle Characteristics Associated With Impaired Balance and Functional Ability in Older People", Hylton B. Menz, Meg E. Morris, and Stephen R. Lord, Journal of Gerontology: MEDICAL SCIENCES, 2005, Vol. 60A, No. 12, 1546–1552

14 Paul Chek, CHEK Institute, www.chekinstitute.com

15 Walter F. Drew, co-founder of the Reusable Resource Association and the Institute for Self Active Education, www.sltrc.com/drdrewstoys.html (January, 2006)

16 Dr. Pauline Camacho, director of Loyola, University's Osteoporosis and Metabolic Bone Disease Center

17 "Dehydration," (January, 2006) MayoClinic.com, www.mayoclinic.com/health/dehydration, (January 18, 2006)

18 Dr. Paul Donohue

19 AARP, "Let's Dance to Health," (January, 2006), www.aarp.org/health (January 20, 2006)

20 "Osteoporosis: A Challenge for Midlife and Older Women," (2005) Older Women League (OWL), www.owl-national.org/osteoporosis.html (January 16, 2006)

21 Neuro-Ophthalmologist Dr. David N. Smith

22 "Calorie Burners: Activities That Turn Up the Heat," (2005), American Council on Exercise, www.acefitness.org/fitfacts (January 25, 2006)

23 Twain, Mark, Quote DB, www.quotedb.com/quotes/2338

Order How To Prevent Falls for a friend today!

**Cut out this page, fill out form on both sides and mail.
Or, buy online today at www.senior-fitness.com.**

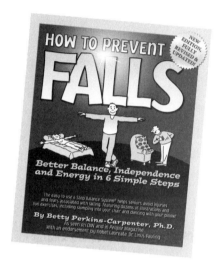

How To Prevent Falls: $16.95 plus $4.50 shipping.
Please send _____ copies of *How To Prevent Falls*

Fill out reverse side with your name and address and send with check or money order to:

**Senior Fitness Productions, Inc.
1780 Penfield Road
Penfield, New York 14526-2104 USA**

Please allow 2-3 weeks for delivery.

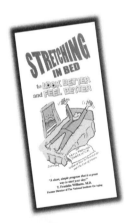

Stretching In Bed: $3.95 plus $1.50 shipping.
Please send _____ copies of *Stretching In Bed*

Fill out reverse side with your name and address and send with check or money order to:

**Senior Fitness Productions, Inc.
1780 Penfield Road
Penfield, New York 14526-2104 USA**

Please allow 2-3 weeks for delivery.

Stretching In Bed is a folded guide of 14 safe stretching exercises designed for use in bed. This guide can stand alone on your night stand. (These exercises are also included in the first chapter of *How To Prevent Falls*.)

Order both & save!

Pay only $18.95, plus $4.50 shipping when you order both *How To Prevent Falls* & the *Stretching In Bed* guide together.

☐ Yes! Please rush me *How To Prevent Falls* and *Stretching In Bed* guide for $23.45 today!

Order Form:

Cut out this page, fill out form on both sides and mail.
Or, buy online today at www.senior-fitness.com.

Name _____

Address _____

City _____ State _____ Zip _____

Payment: ❏ Check   ❏ Money Order   ❏ Credit Card (fill out information below)

Amount Enclosed $ _____ . _____ (NY State residents: Add 8.25% sales tax.)

Credit Card Information

Credit Card Type: ❏ Visa   ❏ MasterCard

Credit Card Account #: _____

Credit Card Expiration Date: ____ /____ /____ Phone: _____

Name as it appears on Credit Card: _____

Payment Amount: $ _____ . _____ (US Dollars)

Cardholder Signature: _____

❏ **Yes!** Please e-mail me important news and information from Senior Fitness, Inc.

E-mail: _____

(Senior Fitness, Inc. will not sell, rent, share or otherwise voluntarily disclose customer e-mail addresses or other identifying information with any third party.)

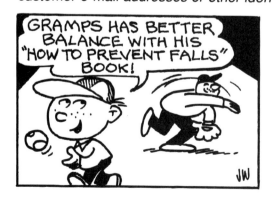

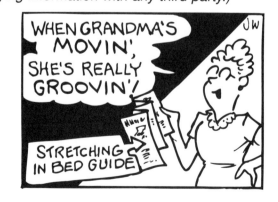